DR. GALEA'S SECRETS TO OPTIMAL HEALTH

Body and Spirit

D1511582

To Carol
Enjoy reading
Dr Galea's secrets!
love Helena

DR. GALEA'S SECRETS TO OPTIMAL HEALTH
Body and Spirit

A simple plan to revitalize body and spirit

- Discover the benefits of balancing hormones
- Learn about homocysteine and how it puts you at risk for heart disease and osteoporosis
- Learn how hormones affect your weight
- Discover why diets fail
- Develop the perfect eating plan for you
- Learn about foods that have a positive affect on your health
- Learn how to stay healthy and youthful with diet
- Learn about Metabolic Syndrome and Inflammation
- Discover how to obtain health benefits from just 30 minutes of exercise a day
- Learn exercises that meet your specific needs
- Learn what causes some of the more common injuries and how to treat them
- Discover how spirituality affects your health

Dr. Anthony Galea M.D.
With Helena Gresik BSc.

Galea, Anthony, 1959–

    Dr. Galea's Secrets to Optimal Health – Body and Spirit/
       Anthony Galea with Helena Gresik

1. Nutrition 2. Aging and hormones 3. Fitness 4. Injuries I. Gresik, Helena. II. Title.

ISBN 978-0-9782659-0-8

This book is intended as a guide and reference book only. It is not meant to substitute for medical advice given to you by your doctor. The authors disclaim liability for any medical outcomes that may occur as a result of recommendations made in this book. Caution is advised in following treatments with hormones, and changes in diet or exercise routines. It is best to consult with your doctor before adopting a new health regime.

Cover Design: Break Point Design, www.breakpointdesign.ca
Text Design, Page Layout and Print Production: WeMakeBooks.ca

11 10 09 08 07   1 2 3 4 5
Printed and bound in Canada

To my cherished wife and soul mate, Nela,
and to the greatest achievement in my life,
my six children, Rachel, Ryan, Brendan,
Madeline, Kaya and Gabriella.

Anthony Galea

Table of Contents

Acknowledgments

We would like to gratefully acknowledge and thank the many friends and colleagues who assisted us in writing this book. We would like to give special thanks to:

- Dr. Tommy Bacher, M.D. and Dr. Keith Pine, M.D. for taking time to edit the manuscript and offer advice.
- Pastor Ralph Rutledge our spiritual advisor and dear friend.
- Dr. Donald M. Carmont for his expert editing of the chapter on Spirituality.
- Mark McCoy for demonstrating the exercises. Mark, the 110 meter hurdles Gold Medal winner at the Barcelona Olympics and the current world record holder for the 50 meter hurdles, is the fitness consultant to Dr. Galea's Institute of Sports Medicine and Wellness Centre in Toronto.

- Noel Mercieca of Break Point Design, Toronto, an exceptional artist and illustrator, for the artwork, cover design and photography that was used in our book.
- Heidy Lawrance and her staff at Heidy Lawrance Associates for their expert assistance in preparing our book for publishing.
- Helena would like to thank Linda Mikus for her comments and advice in writing the chapter on Spirituality.
- Special thanks to Rob Patterson for the countless hours he spent proofreading the manuscript while it was being written.

Introduction

I am 47 years old, have six children, am a sports medicine doctor with an extremely busy practice and travel extensively for my job. I'm passionate about sports, cycling, skiing, snow-boarding, and I want to be able to participate in these activities for many years to come. I enjoy the full, active and balanced life that I have. I want to stay healthy and active well into my senior years, and I want to motivate you to improve your quality of life so you can stay healthy and active well into your senior years too. This is why I wrote this book.

Over the past few years, there has been an alarming increase in obesity and in diseases strongly influenced by diet, such as type 2 diabetes and heart disease. I believe that part of the reason for this increase is that many people are simply unaware of how important it is to keep hormones in balance and the critical role that food plays in hormone control and health.

It is always better to prevent a disease than it is to cure it. Diseases such as type 2 diabetes and heart disease can be prevented in many cases just by improving our diet and being more active. To understand this connection, you must first understand how hormones function.

In Part I of this book, I have discussed a number of the major hormones, such as insulin, glucagon and cortisol, and the effects that they have on health and aging. I've discussed the benefits and cautions of hormone replacement. If you are considering hormone replacement, you should be aware of bioidentical hormones and significant hormones such as growth hormone, progesterone, estrogen, testosterone, melatonin and DHEA. It is important to understand how these hormones affect your wellness.

In Part II, I have discussed metabolic syndrome and inflammation, which both negatively affect health and which may be controlled with the foods we eat. I have discussed some of the more popular weight loss diets, healthy foods and my Perfect Eating Plan. This plan will give you the nutrients you need to keep your hormones in balance and keep you healthy, slim, vibrant and youthful.

Many people, who are struggling with weight control, often cringe at the thought of the excessive amount of exercise required to stay slim and healthy. In Part III, I have detailed an exercise plan that does not have to take more than 30 minutes a day, four or five times a week. You don't have to follow the exercise schedule of an athlete to attain health benefits. Many times, fitness instructors will give people schedules that are so grueling they just can't keep up. They quickly become discouraged and stop exercising. I have concisely described exercises that are not overwhelming, but that will keep your core, cardiovascular system and muscles conditioned.

In Part IV, I have described some of the more common injuries, how to prevent them and how to treat them. I have reviewed some of the procedures and medical instrumentation that I have developed to diagnose and treat injuries. The information is easy to read and to follow.

I believe a book on optimal health would not be complete unless our spiritual well-being is addressed. We cannot be totally healthy and happy unless we acknowledge our spirit and encourage it to grow. Hormones, nutrition and exercise address our mind and body, but humans are a three part entity. We consist of mind, body and spirit. We cannot ignore this third part of our makeup – our spirit. Our spirit is the essence of who we are. I have shared with you my own spiritual journey and how it has positively affected my life.

In over 20 years as a sports medicine doctor for numerous professional and Olympic athletes, I have had the privilege to work with many renowned medical specialists, coaches, athletic nutritionists and exercise scientists from around the world. To provide my athletes and patients with the best and most current care, it is essential for me to keep expanding my knowledge of medicine and embracing new techniques. I would like to share this expertise and knowledge with you. I hope you will find *Dr. Galea's Secrets to Optimal Health – Body and Spirit* informative, easy to read and easy to follow on your way to optimal health.

Part I

HORMONES AND BLOOD CHEMISTRY

CHAPTER 1

What Are Hormones?

Hormones are messengers that are made at specific sites in our body, such as the pancreas and the adrenal glands. They are sent out through the bloodstream to stimulate specific actions, such as stabilizing our blood glucose levels or controlling the amount of body fat that we produce and store. Without the correct amount of hormones, be it too little or too much, our bodies don't get the proper direction and we become more susceptible to disease. Keeping hormones in balance is one of the most important factors in the prevention of premature aging.

This may seem like a daunting task as there are many hormones that give our bodies direction. Insulin, glucagon, cortisol, testosterone, progesterone, estrogen, DHEA, growth hormone and adrenaline are a few of the hormones our body produces in order to function on a daily basis. Each hormone is programmed for a particular function and without the right amount of this hormone, our bodies will not perform optimally. We may feel tired, sluggish, not at our best and this may occur for a number of years before a more serious condition develops.

Our hormone system is complex and intricate. Sometimes several hormones can affect one function – for instance, blood glucose is affected by the hormones insulin, glucagon, and cortisol. Other times, one hormone can affect several functions – for example, insulin can affect our blood glucose levels, the amount of body fat we store, and the amount of cholesterol the liver produces.

Hormones can interact with each other, so high levels of one hormone can affect another hormone – for example high levels of cortisol can decrease the level of testosterone. Each hormone has a special way of communicating with the particular site that it is meant to maintain and just the right amount of hormone must be present. If this communication fails, or if the hormones are not within the proper range, our feeling of well-being is compromised.

Aging and Hormones

Baby boomers are more than a little interested in staying healthy and vibrant as they age. They want to stay active physically and continue to look youthful and healthy as they grow older. They want to look and feel at least a decade younger so that "sixty is the new fifty". The boomer generation is economically and socially powerful. Because of their interest in staying healthy and active, much discussion has taken place and many studies have been done on hormones and how they affect our health.

Many of our hormones, such as growth hormone, testosterone and estrogen decrease dramatically with age, while others, such as dihydrotestosterone and insulin, increase. Time and time again research points to the fact that we will be burdened with diseases that affect the aged if our hormones are not kept in balance.

It is not only the baby boom generation that should be interested in hormones. More and more young people in their teens and twenties have high insulin levels and are being diagnosed with type 2 diabetes – a disease that was previously affecting middle aged individuals. Every age group should be concerned with their hormone levels. Often correct hormone balance can be achieved with only an adjustment to our diet and the amount of exercise we get.

We need to take control of our health and take a more individualized approach to our health issues. Sometimes, people accept "feeling out of sorts" as part of the aging process. They feel this way for years not knowing that changing hormone levels are the culprit to their malaise and that their vitality could be restored by simply adjusting these levels.

Not all family doctors have caught up to the research on hormones. Some doctors would like us to believe that these changes are just part of the normal aging process. It is essential for our health and well-being to search out a physician who is knowledgeable and is willing to do the regular testing required to keep our hormones in the correct range.

Each person's blood chemistry is unique and needs to be tested in order to evaluate the proper course of action. Two people of the same age could have very different blood chemistry. We need to stay informed and involved with our health issues. Many diseases could be prevented by keeping our hormones in a healthy range rather than being given numerous prescription drugs to treat symptoms after years of improper hormone balance.

Bioidentical Hormones

Hormone control can be achieved with proper diet, exercise, avoiding stress, eliminating smoking and avoiding chemicals. If necessary, bioidentical hormones can be used to replace the natural hormones that we lose as we age. Bioidentical hormones are not synthetic hormones and do not have the same side effects. They are more likely to mimic the natural hormones that we have lost. Unfortunately, not all doctors are familiar with bioidentical hormones and will not prescribe them but will steer you toward drugs and synthetic hormones.

As an example, some doctors will prescribe the synthetic estrogen/progestin combination to women experiencing menopausal symptoms without doing a blood test. A test of hormone levels would determine if the woman requires more estrogen or if progesterone on its own would be enough to balance her hormones. Doctors are prescribing on the studies and recommendations made by pharmaceutical companies. They don't have time to research each drug that comes on the market so most doctors are influenced by information provided by these companies.

The synthetic estrogen/progestin combination is patentable and therefore profitable while bioidentical progesterone is not. Pharmaceutical companies provide doctors not only with literature, but also with free samples to dispense to their patients.

Bioidentical estrogen and progesterone are synthesized from plant extracts such as yams and soybeans. They are designed molecularly to be similar to the hormones in our bodies. These hormones have been used in Europe for many years with great success and minimal side effects.

Drugs can be important for our medical care and they do save lives, but often we are given drugs to alleviate symptoms when we only require a change in our diet and a tweaking of our blood chemistry.

Should Hormones Be Replaced?

It is important to find a knowledgeable doctor who is willing to do the necessary tests to determine your hormone levels before giving you a prescription. Your doctor should also be interested and involved in helping you keep your hormones properly adjusted in the years to come. Each person's blood chemistry is unique and keeps changing with age. Replacing our hormones when needed and keeping the hormone levels in control is an important part of our health care.

Mainstream medicine can take years to catch up with research. For many years now, significant research has been carried out on balancing hormones. The findings of these studies have indicated positive effects on health and wellness. However, some doctors are wary of the information or do not have time or an interest in finding out about these new medical treatments. It is important to explore new knowledge and benefit from it. In the 1950's, cholesterol testing was just in its infancy. Now, it has been used for years to flag potential heart problems and is completely accepted by the medical profession.

It is crucial to your health to find a physician who is familiar with the benefits of balancing hormones and who can monitor your progress if you decide to replace hormones. There are many doctors who keep in touch with current technology and embrace it. It is interesting to note that physicians were among the first to supplement with growth hormone. Keeping hormones in the proper range can improve the quality of a person's life as well as ward off disease.

Understanding the function and importance of some of our major hormones and how vital it is to keep them in control will allow us to make a more informed decision regarding our own health.

CHAPTER 2

Insulin and Glucagon

INSULIN

Most of us have heard of insulin, but only a few of us are aware of how significant it is to our health. Insulin is a powerful hormone and it is critical to keep the right balance of insulin in our bloodstream to optimally maintain our health. It is produced by the pancreas and it takes glucose from our bloodstream and moves it into our cells. Once inside the cells, glucose can be used immediately for energy or stored for future use. Insulin has the key to unlock the cells and deliver the glucose; without insulin our cells would starve.

As we age, insulin levels tend to increase and this rapidly accelerates the aging process. An excessive amount of insulin for an extended period of time can disrupt many other hormone systems in our body which can lead to disease. High insulin levels can increase the risk of:

- **High cholesterol**
- **Stroke**
- **Excessive body fat.** Insulin causes fat to be stored in our body. An excess of insulin will prevent the release of body fat from our cells. If insulin levels are stabilized, the stored body fat is released and used for energy during the day.
- **Fat deposits in the lining of the arteries.** These deposits can cause high blood pressure and eventually clogged arteries.
- **Inflammation.** High levels of insulin create chemicals in the body that can result in inflammation and this inflammation can eventually result in visible aging of the skin. Recent studies have shown that inflammation can also cause more serious degenerative diseases such as heart disease, cancer and Alzheimer's. I will discuss these studies in the chapter on inflammation.
- **Premature aging**

For us to remain youthful and healthy, insulin is the single most important hormone to keep in balance.

What Is Insulin Resistance?

Insulin resistance occurs when the normal amount of insulin can't open the cells to transfer the glucose from the bloodstream into the cells. In an effort to maintain a normal amount of glucose in the blood, the pancreas then produces more insulin to try to force the glucose into the cells. If this increased insulin can't transfer the glucose into the cells, then high amounts of glucose remain in the bloodstream and type 2 diabetes occurs. Insulin resistance is common in people who are obese or who have cardiovascular disease or high blood pressure.

How Can You Tell If You Have Elevated Insulin Levels?

Have your blood tested for fasting insulin, triglycerides and cholesterol. Excess insulin stimulates the liver to produce more cholesterol. If you are producing too much insulin, you are more at risk for heart disease and other degenerative diseases. We often are not aware that we have elevated insulin levels and we could go on experiencing symptoms such as increased fat levels, high blood pressure and high cholesterol, not knowing the cause. This is why we need to take control of our health and have the necessary tests done to ensure that our hormones stay in a healthy range.

Low Insulin Levels

Insulin levels can also be too low. The type 1 diabetic is unable to make insulin and must take insulin injections daily or their cells would starve as they have no way of taking glucose from their blood to feed their cells without insulin. Only a small percentage of diabetics are type 1.

Most people who have diabetes are type 2 diabetics; their bodies have produced too much insulin and they have become insulin resistant. The insulin they produce can no longer move the glucose into the cells and high amounts of glucose remain in the blood.

It is possible by eating a high protein, low carbohydrate diet to push your insulin levels too low. If insulin levels are too low, you could develop low blood pressure, loss of muscle tissue, fatigue, irritability, increased hunger and ketosis. Ketosis is a condition where there is an excess of ketones in the body. This is caused when insulin levels drop and the glycogen in the liver is depleted trying to restore glucose levels. The body then begins to break down fats leaving behind a by-product called ketones. Low carbohydrate diets encourage the breakdown of fat and can induce dietary ketosis, which is not a healthy condition.

It is important to note that health risks increase when the levels of insulin are too high as well as when the levels of insulin are too low. It is critical to keep this hormone in balance.

How Do You Keep Insulin Levels Balanced?

In most cases, diet and exercise can keep insulin levels controlled. Diet has more effect on our insulin levels than exercise, but the combination of proper diet and exercise is the best way to keep insulin levels in balance.

- Aerobic exercise lowers both blood glucose and insulin levels.
- Insulin is very much affected by the food we eat. A meal, containing one third of the plate as protein and two thirds of the plate as vegetables and fruit, would be an ideal meal to control insulin levels. It is also essential to eat a small amount of a healthy fat at each meal, such as walnuts, cashews, avocado or olive oil.

Fats slow down the entry of carbohydrates into the bloodstream so less insulin is produced when some fat is eaten with a meal or snack.

■ Not skipping meals and eating breakfast, lunch and dinner plus two small snacks throughout the day controls insulin levels. I will discuss this in more detail in the chapter on diet and nutrition.

■ Carbohydrates with a high glycemic index should be avoided as much as possible. Soft drinks, processed foods, chips, cakes, cookies and white flour should be avoided or severely limited.

What Is Glycemic Index?

The glycemic index is a measure of how fast a carbohydrate enters the bloodstream as glucose. The higher the glycemic index, the more insulin is produced by our body. Fruits and vegetables usually have a low glycemic index. Breads, potatoes, and rice have high glycemic indices. It's important to know the actual glycemic index of carbohydrates because not all is as it seems. Most people would consider table sugar as having the highest glycemic index of all. In fact, sugar is actually lower than rice, potatoes and bread. If these foods are kept to a minimum in our diet then insulin levels will be controlled more easily.

GLUCAGON

Many people have heard about insulin, but the hormone glucagon, which works in conjunction with insulin, is a relative unknown. Insulin and glucagon are the two hormones that work together to maintain the level of blood glucose in the tight range that our body requires. Glucagon is a hormone secreted by the pancreas and its main function is to release stored glucose from the liver into the bloodstream when glucose levels drop too low.

If glucose levels increase in our bloodstream, then insulin is secreted by the pancreas to carry and deposit glucose into our cells. This lowers the level of glucose in our bloodstream.

If glucose levels in our bloodstream are too low, such as when we are exercising or have not eaten for a while, glucagon is secreted by the pancreas to release stored glucose from the liver into the bloodstream.

Insulin and glucagon must always be in proper balance. When one hormone goes up, the other goes down. Carbohydrates stimulate the release of insulin. Dietary protein stimulates the release of glucagon. Without adequate levels of glucagon you will feel hungry and tired because you are not getting enough fuel. If we eat a proper balance of protein to carbohydrate at every meal and snack we can keep glucagon and insulin in balance, and when these two hormones are in balance, blood glucose is stabilized and our body will perform optimally.

Your glucose levels should be tested yearly. Fasting blood glucose levels should be maintained in the proper range. If you are producing excess glucose, you are considered to be hyperglycemic and if you have insufficient glucose in your bloodstream, you are considered to be hypoglycemic. Keeping glucose in the healthy range is imperative to your health and to avoid age–related diseases.

CHAPTER 3

Cortisol

Cortisol is considered to be one of our major hormones. Often it is called the stress hormone because this is the hormone released by the body in response to stressful situations. Cortisol is produced in the adrenal glands which are small glands located adjacent to the kidneys.

Cortisol is secreted during stressful situations such as:

- trauma
- excessive exercise
- temperature variations
- lack of sleep
- poor eating habits
- attacks on our body by viruses and bacteria

- emotional stress brought on by financial, job, or family pressures

A little stress is good for the body because it stimulates the adrenal glands to produce cortisol. Our bodies need cortisol to be able to cope with stressful situations. Without some stress, the adrenal glands would begin to atrophy and reduce production of cortisol.

But too much stress is not a good situation. If our bodies remain under constant stress for long periods of time without the opportunity to recover, the adrenal glands produce excessive amounts of cortisol, become overworked and eventually, burn out. Cortisol production is stopped.

It is important to keep this hormone in balance. Cortisol levels that are too low can cause us to become irritable, lethargic and extremely fatigued. Cortisol levels that are too high for extended periods of time can cause:

- Our body to age at an accelerated rate
- Breakdown of muscle protein so muscle mass and strength is lost.
- Bone loss and osteoporosis
- Suppression of the immune system
- Heart disease

- Damage to brain cells
- Storage of abdominal fat

When faced with stressful situations our bodies secrete cortisol to fight off the dangers. Cortisol increases the flow of glucose, protein and fat from our cells into the bloodstream. This provides energy to our body to cope with the stress. This is a good thing for a stressful situation that is resolved immediately, but if the stress continues for a long time then glucose is constantly being fed into our bloodstream, and more insulin is produced to deal with the added glucose.

If the cortisol levels and insulin levels remain high, we become insulin resistant and have all the problems that are associated with insulin resistance, such as accumulation of abdominal fat, inflammation and high cholesterol. Also, with high cortisol levels, protein continues to be removed from our muscles and muscle mass and strength are lost.

Cortisol is important to our well-being. We need our adrenal glands to be able to produce cortisol, but too much or too little cortisol can cause problems. Once again, as with the other hormones we have already discussed, cortisol must be kept within range in order for us to function at our full potential.

How Do You Keep Cortisol at a Safe Level?

- **Stress reduction.** Meditation, deep breathing or relaxing with your favourite book or hobby are ways to reduce emotional stress.
- **Moderate exercise.** Intense exercise is not recommended as it can actually increase stress and cortisol levels. Working out for 30 to 45 minutes a day should give you a sufficient amount of exercise without increasing cortisol levels excessively.
- **Proper diet.** It is important to get an appropriate amount of protein, carbohydrate and fat at each meal to keep insulin, glucagon and cortisol in balance.

What Are Your Cortisol Levels?

Blood tests can determine cortisol levels. Cortisol levels in the blood are the highest between three and six o'clock in the morning. This is to deal with the stress of the overnight fast. Cortisol gradually decreases during the day. This rise and fall of cortisol is normal and important to our health. A blood test to determine cortisol levels should be done in the morning after fasting and another blood sample should be drawn in the late afternoon.

CHAPTER 4

Testosterone and Dihydrotestosterone (DHT)

TESTOSTERONE

Testosterone is usually considered a male hormone and estrogen a female hormone. In actual fact, both hormones are produced by both sexes. The difference is that men produce significantly more testosterone than women and women produce more estrogen than men.

In males, testosterone is a sex hormone produced in the testes and is responsible for a man's facial hair, his baldness and his deep voice. Testosterone:

- increases libido

- helps develop muscle mass and strength
- stimulates the production of sperm

As men begin to age, their testosterone levels drop and by age 50, testosterone levels could be up to 50% less than at age 25. This phase in a man's life is called andropause, the male equivalent of menopause. The hormonal change in andropause can be an increase in the level of estrogen as well as a decrease in the level testosterone. It is very important to have hormone levels tested in order to determine the correct course of action.

In menopause, some women experience noticeable and unbearable symptoms as hormone levels drop quickly and dramatically. With men, hormone changes are gradual and could occur over a 10 year period, so the symptoms they experience are not as noticeable. Men lose energy, ambition and sex drive gradually over time. These changes are often attributed to burnout or depression rather than low testosterone levels. Low levels of testosterone are associated with:

- impotence
- decreased libido
- the accumulation of body fat
- loss of lean body mass

- loss of strength and energy
- increased risk of osteoporosis
- loss of short-term memory
- fatigue
- irritability
- depression

Maintaining Levels of Testosterone

Maintaining proper levels of testosterone as a man ages is closely tied to proper diet, exercise and stress control.

- Testosterone levels decline and estrogen levels increase with an increase in body fat. It is important to eat a diet that keeps insulin levels in check to prevent excess body fat. The more stored body fat a man has, the more testosterone is converted into estrogen.
- The mineral zinc and vitamin C inhibit the enzyme aromatase that converts testosterone to estrogen. A deficiency in zinc and/or vitamin C will result in higher levels of estrogen and lower levels of testosterone.
- Anaerobic exercise, such as weight training, increases testosterone in both men and women and should be

part of your program to maintain testosterone levels. However, intense weight training should be avoided as cortisol levels begin to increase after about 45 minutes of weight training. High cortisol levels decrease the levels of testosterone.

- All types of stress, not only intense anaerobic exercise, will increase cortisol levels. The more you can reduce the various stresses in your life, the less cortisol will be circulating in your bloodstream and the more testosterone will remain.

Men who are middle aged and are missing their usual energy and vitality, have a decreased libido and are sleeping more than usual, especially during the day, should consider having their testosterone levels tested. Usually, the blood work that is done during a regular yearly physical exam does not include testing for this hormone.

Replacing Testosterone in Men

Hormone replacement is not considered by many family physicians as an important consideration in the health and well-being of the patient. It has always been a well known fact that hormones, inevitably, decline with age, but not until recently did some doctors consider replacing the lost hormones to improve the wellness of their patients.

If testosterone levels are low, replacing the lost testosterone with bioidentical testosterone can improve vitality, vigor and the sense of well-being. It is important to work with a competent physician who can first determine if you are a candidate for testosterone replacement. If you are, your physician must then determine the proper dosage that you would require and carefully monitor your progress during treatment.

Each individual should make the decision for himself. He should consider the risks and the benefits. Bioidentical testosterone can be replaced in pill form, with transdermal preparations such as a patch or gel, or by injection.

Benefits of Replacing Testosterone in Men

- prevent osteoporosis and maintain bone density
- restore muscle strength and develop muscle mass
- improve mental acuity
- improve vitality
- increase libido
- restore sexual functioning

Cautions of Replacing Testosterone in Men

- may increase risk of prostate cancer and breast cancer
- may increase levels of triglycerides and cholesterol; caution is advised when supplementing testosterone in men with significant risk factors for cardiovascular disease
- may cause negative behavioral patterns
- may worsen sleep apnea

If I replace testosterone in a male patient, for the first six months I do blood tests monthly and then one every three months. I test for an increase in lipids, DHT, liver enzymes, PSA (prostate-specific antigen) and hemoglobin. If your testosterone levels are low and you chose to replace this hormone, then you should be under the care of a knowl-edgeable physician and be monitored carefully during treatment.

Replacing Testosterone in Women

In females, testosterone is made in the ovaries and adrenal glands. Testosterone levels are usually highest in women in their twenties and then begin to drop until menopause when the ovaries drastically reduce the production of all sex hormones.

Low testosterone levels can decrease libido. Testosterone vaginal creams can relieve vaginal dryness, act as a lubricant, and increase sex drive. When using testosterone, the dose should be monitored carefully. Too much testosterone can cause the growth of facial hair, the loss of hair on your head, oily skin, acne, a deepened voice, an aggressive personality, risk of heart and liver disease.

Benefits of Replacing Testosterone in Women

- increases libido
- relieves vaginal dryness
- increases sense of well–being
- improves muscle mass and strength

Cautions of Replacing Testosterone in Women

- may increase cholesterol levels
- may increase risk of heart disease
- may increase risk of liver disease
- may increase growth of facial hair

■ may cause a more aggressive personality

It is important to consult with your physician to determine if your testosterone levels are low and if you would benefit from replacing this hormone. If you do chose to replace testosterone then you should be under the care of a knowledgeable physician and be monitored carefully during treatment as dosage might have to be adjusted often to get the proper balance. Bioidentical testosterone is available in gel, drops, cream and capsule form.

DIHYDROTESTOSTERONE (DHT)

Dihydrotestosterone (DHT), a by-product of testosterone, is a powerful form of testosterone and is associated with prostate enlargement and male pattern baldness. Testosterone is converted to the more potent form, DHT, within the prostate gland. As a man ages, the production of DHT increases and this causes the cells of the prostate to divide and multiply at a faster rate, leading to an enlarged prostate.

Men with an enlarged prostate will notice an increased frequency of urination, reduced urine stream and the need to urinate frequently during the night. There is a strong link between high levels of DHT and prostate cancer.

As a man ages, his body makes less testosterone, however, the prostate gland more aggressively converts the available testosterone to DHT. This is due to the enzyme 5-alpha-reductase, which converts testosterone to DHT in the prostate and which becomes more active with age. Approximately 50 to 60% of men between 40 and 59 years of age develop an enlarged prostate gland.

Saw Palmetto Berries and DHT

Research has shown that saw palmetto berries contain active ingredients that naturally inhibit the 5-alpha-reductase enzyme. However, saw palmetto berries on their own are not effective as they only have 1.5% fatty acids and sterols. To be effective, saw palmetto extracts must be made and standardized to contain 85 to 95% fatty acids and sterols.

In this form, they may also block the conversion of testosterone into estrogen. Estrogen inhibits the breakdown of DHT in the prostate and, therefore, contributes to prostate enlargement.

However, recent studies, published in the February 2006 issue of the *New England Journal of Medicine*, found no significant difference between a saw palmetto pill and a placebo in men with moderate to advanced prostate problems. In the past, at least 20 trials with saw palmetto showed positive outcomes. None of the studies that have been done to date show any significant side effects or toxicity related to saw palmetto extract.

Since there is still some debate on this subject, it may be beneficial for men with high levels of DHT or men taking testosterone or DHEA replacement to also add saw palmetto to their regimens. If they see no significant reduction in their DHT levels, then their doctors can prescribe finasteride. However, this drug may have side effects, including erectile difficulties and a lowered sex drive.

It is strongly recommended that men over 40 years old have their levels of DHT tested by their physicians.

CHAPTER 5

Estrogen and Progesterone

Estrogen, like testosterone, is produced by both men and women, but women have much more estrogen than men. In women, estrogen works together with progesterone to nourish and support the female reproductive tissues and breasts. There are three estrogens that are primarily produced by the ovaries but are also produced in smaller quantities by other tissues such as the liver, adrenal glands, breasts and body fat. Progesterone is secreted by the ovary during the last two weeks of the menstrual cycle.

The three estrogens made by the female body are:

- estrone

- estradiol
- estriol

These three estrogens are not always at the same concentrations, but they vary during the month and during pregnancy.

Estradiol is the most powerful of the three estrogens and this is the one that promotes breast cancer. Estriol, on the other hand, is significantly less powerful than estradiol and some studies show that estriol may actually protect against breast cancer.

Monthly Cycle of Estrogen and Progesterone in Women

The level of estrogen and progesterone varies during different stages of the menstrual cycle.

- Estradiol is the primary estrogen produced during the first two weeks of a woman's menstrual cycle. It is at its highest concentration at mid cycle.
- Estradiol levels peak just prior to ovulation and then drop off drastically. It is this sharp drop of estradiol that triggers the ovulation process.

- After ovulation, progesterone and estrogen levels start to rise. The progesterone levels will now be twice as high as the estrogen.

- As progesterone increases, estradiol is converted into estrone and then into estriol, therefore, estriol is at its highest level at this point in the cycle.

- If there is no pregnancy, then estrogen and progesterone levels fall abruptly triggering the shedding of the lining of the uterus and menstruation begins.

- If a woman is pregnant, then estriol is made in large quantities and estrone levels increase, but estradiol levels are the lowest at this time. Progesterone levels increase, and with the higher levels of progesterone, the lining of the uterus remains intact and does not shed. As pregnancy progresses, progesterone continues to be produced by the placenta for the duration of the pregnancy.

Perimenopause

As a woman ages, the balance of estrogen and progesterone begins to shift. It is this balance that is even more important than the levels of the individual hormones. Many women stop ovulating in their early forties but continue to menstruate. If a woman stops ovulating, she will also stop producing progesterone, but she could still be producing estrogen.

Without progesterone, she will have a hormonal imbalance and can begin experiencing menopausal symptoms. She could continue to produce estrogen and have periods for the next decade but experience the unpleasant symptoms of menopause because of a lack of progesterone. At this point, she is said to be in perimenopause.

Perimenopause does not mean that a woman has excessive estrogen, it just means that her estrogen level is higher than normal compared to the progesterone level so the hormones are not in proper balance. In perimenopause:

- A woman could experience regular or irregular menstrual cycles. She could have heavy bleeding some months and miss her period for a month or two as her estrogen production becomes erratic producing high levels one month and low levels the next.
- Estrogen dominance occurs because estrogen is being produced and progesterone is not.
- With estrogen dominance, some women could experience menopausal symptoms such as moodiness, water retention, sore and swollen breasts, difficulty sleeping and weight gain. This could go on for many years

before estrogen levels drop completely putting a halt to menstruation.

It is necessary to have both estrogen and progesterone levels measured in order that the proper course of action can be taken. If a woman's estrogen levels are in the proper range, but the progesterone levels are low, then replacing progesterone with bioidentical progesterone can reverse the symptoms of perimenopause. It is important to balance the hormones and replace only the hormone that is deficient.

Some doctors will prescribe a synthetic combination of estrogen and progestin without doing blood tests to determine hormone levels. A woman will then be receiving even more estrogen along with the synthetic progestin, and although this could ease some of the symptoms of perimenopause, it could create other problems. Studies have shown that women using the combination estrogen and synthetic progestin therapy, have had an increased incidence of breast cancer and heart disease.

Menopause

Menopause occurs when the ovaries stop producing estrogen and menstruation ceases. Menopause is diagnosed officially

43

when a woman has not been menstruating for a year. Some women may have very few symptoms during menopause while others may have unbearable symptoms such as:

- hot flashes
- night sweats
- depression
- vaginal dryness
- moodiness
- loss of sex drive
- an itching of the skin or scalp
- inability to sleep through the night

In most cases, these symptoms can be alleviated by balancing a woman's hormone levels. This is not an easy task as every woman is unique and will have a different requirement.

If you consider replacing estrogen and progesterone, it is best to replace with the smallest amount that will alleviate menopausal symptoms. Some women may only need natural progesterone cream; others may require both estrogen and progesterone. Have your doctor do the necessary blood test to determine your hormone levels before you start treatment. Your doctor should continue to monitor your hormones regularly, as your hormone levels will change. It may be necessary to adjust your dosage to maintain the correct balance. You should not be taking hormones without medical supervision and it is imperative to find a physician who is familiar with bioidentical hormone replacement.

The Women's Health Initiative Study (WHI), considered the first ever long term controlled clinical trial of hormone replacement therapy, was halted three years early. Results indicated that the estrogen and progestin combination increased the risk of breast cancer, heart attack, blood clots and stroke. Over 16,000 U.S. women participated in the study that was stopped after five years as the risks exceeded the benefits. The study was intended to run until 2005, but was ended in July 2002. The findings were published in the July 17, 2002 issue of *Journal of the Medical Association.*

The estrogen and progestin used in this study was Premarin (conjugated equine estrogens) and Provera (medroxyprogesterone acetate). Premarin is derived from pregnant horses' urine and contains mostly estrone and a number of horse estrogens that are not natural to humans. Provera is a synthetic progestin. This is the same drug that is used in the morning after pill that is taken to prevent pregnancy. Some studies indicate that it may be the progestin that increases the risk of breast cancer, heart attack and stroke. Natural progesterone is more like the progesterone that the body produces. It is available as a cream or as micronized progesterone, which is taken orally.

The Postmenopausal Estrogen/Progestin Interventions (PEPI) Trial followed 875 postmenopausal women who received one of Premarin, Premarin and Provera, Premarin and micronized progesterone (natural progesterone), or a placebo. Results were published in the *Journal of the American Medical Association* in 1995. Results showed the HDL "good" cholesterol increased by 9% in women taking the regime with micronized progesterone and only 3 to 4% in the women taking Premarin and Provera. PEPI trial investigator Bernadine P. Healy M.D. commented, "I think the biggest surprise certainly was the HDL effect of micronized progesterone." Elizabeth Barret-Connor, cardiologist and PEPI investigator, said: "If I were treating a woman primarily because she was worried about heart disease or because she had dyslipidemia and low HDL cholesterol, I would probably see if she wanted to take micronized (natural) progesterone. I was quite impressed with the better effect."

Dr. Fitzpatrick, from the department of Internal Medicine at the Mayo Clinic, did a review of micronized progesterone and synthetic progesterone. The review, "Micronized Progesterone: Clinical Implications and Comparison with Current Treatments," was published in *Fertility and Sterility*. The author said, "A large body of evidence, including the Postmenopausal Estrogen/Progestin Interventions study suggests that the use of combination estrogen and oral micronized progesterone is optimal for long term hormone replacement therapy." The review indicated that synthetic progestins are associated with many potential negative reactions and that care should be taken in administering these drugs, especially to women in their first trimester of pregnancy, who have high blood pressure or who have diabetes.

Bioidentical Hormones

It is best to achieve hormonal balance with biologically identical hormones as they appear to have far fewer side effects than synthetic drugs. Bioidentical hormones are not as readily available as synthetic hormones because drug companies cannot patent a natural product and make huge profits from it. However, many doctors are becoming more aware of the benefits of natural hormones and are prescribing them. As a result, compounding pharmacies are now available and are making natural bioidentical estrogen and progesterone at varying concentrations.

Bioidentical estradiol, estrone, estriol and progesterone are synthesized from plant extracts such as yams and soybeans. They are designed molecularly to be similar to the hormones in our bodies. Bioidentical hormones have been used in Europe for many years with great success and minimal side effects.

Bioidentical Progesterone

Many menopausal symptoms are reversed with progesterone cream alone. Dr. John Lee has done many years of research on progesterone and has written several books on menopause, including the book *What Your Doctor May Not Tell You About Menopause: The Breakthrough Book on Natural Progesterone*. He has prescribed only natural progesterone to most of his patients. He writes, "My experience, and the experience of many of the doctors who correspond with or call me, has been that most menopausal symptoms will respond to progesterone supplementation alone."

Although progesterone creams are available without prescription, it is recommended to consult with your doctor before using these. Blood tests need to be done to determine the correct dosage you might require. Not all progesterone creams that are available without prescription have the required amount of progesterone in them to make a difference to symptoms. Compounding pharmacies are now making bioidentical progesterone creams in varying concentrations. Once your doctor determines the amount of progesterone you require, a prescription can be written for the correct dosage.

Bioidentical progesterone has been used for years in European countries to alleviate menopausal symptoms. It is now also available in a micronized form, which is taken orally. Progesterone is best taken at bedtime, as it can make some women drowsy.

Bioidentical progesterone protects against endometrial cancer as well as breast cancer, is a natural diuretic and helps build bone making it protective against osteoporosis. If a woman is experiencing vaginal dryness leading to vaginal and bladder infections, progesterone cream alone may help with these symptoms.

Estriol Vaginal Cream

If vaginal dryness cannot be alleviated with progesterone cream, then a vaginal application of a natural bioidentical estriol cream used twice a week may solve the problem. Even though estriol is the weakest of the estrogens, it is found to be most effective on vaginal tissue. It is also the least likely to be implicated in causing cancer.

Benefits of Replacing Estrogen and Progesterone

- reduces the risk of osteoporosis by preserving bone mass

- may reduce the risk of colon cancer
- improves sense of well-being
- improves sleep
- improves memory

Cautions of Replacing Estrogen and Progesterone

- may increase risk of breast cancer
- may increase risk of blood clots
- may increase risk of cardiovascular disease
- may increase risk of gall bladder disease
- may increase risk of high blood pressure in some women

I am prescribing only bioidentical progesterone to patients who have sufficient estrogen, and bioidentical estrogen and progesterone to others who are lacking both estrogen and progesterone. It is essential to be under a doctor's care if you decide to replace these hormones. Regular blood tests should be done to check hormone levels and make adjustments when necessary to maintain the correct balance.

CHAPTER 6

Dehydroepiandrosterone and Melatonin

DEHYDROEPIANDROSTERONE (DHEA)

DHEA (dehydroepiandrosterone) is a steroid hormone primarily made from cholesterol in the adrenal glands and is also made by the brain and skin in smaller amounts. It is the most abundant steroid hormone produced by the body. DHEA levels in the blood peak at around age 20 and then gradually decline. At age 65 your body makes only about 15% of the amount it made at age 20. DHEA is involved in the production of testosterone, estrogen and progesterone.

It has long been considered an anti-aging hormone because levels drop significantly as we age and many diseases of old age correlate with low levels of DHEA.

Benefits of Replacing DHEA

- **May decrease body fat.** Arthur Schwartz, PhD, of the Fells Institute for Cancer Research and Molecular Biology at Temple University, has done much research on DHEA. He administered DHEA to mice and found that four out of five mice lost 31% body fat while their weight stayed the same. The results were identical in a study done with humans, which showed that high doses of DHEA caused a decrease in body fat and an increase in muscle mass in four out of five subjects. DHEA seems to inhibit an enzyme which interferes with the body's ability to store fat and it also signals the body to feel full. Studies done by Samuel Yen, professor of reproductive studies at the University Of California School Of Medicine, showed that fat mass decreased in men but not in women.
- **May improve the immune system and sense of well-being.** A three month study done by Samuel

Yen showed that administering 50 mg of DHEA to 71 women and 13 men between the ages of 40 and 70 resulted in both men and women reporting an improved sense of well-being. Furthermore, researchers found that the immune system was enhanced with the increased level of DHEA.

■ **DHEA may reduce risk of heart disease in men but not in women.** In 1995, studies done by Elizabeth Barrett–Connor at the University of California, San Diego showed a 15% drop in deaths from heart disease in men with higher levels of DHEA. This was not the case with women, as the same study showed there was no association between heart disease and levels of DHEA in women. An earlier study in 1986, done by the same group of researchers, reported that men with high levels of DHEA were far less likely to die of heart disease while women with high levels of DHEA were at greater risk.

Cautions of Replacing DHEA

■ This hormone should be used with caution by women, especially postmenopausal women. Some studies indicated that although high levels of DHEA in pre-menopausal women showed lower incidence of cancer, the opposite was true with postmenopausal women. Also, in postmenopausal women, higher DHEA levels are associated with weight gain and insulin resistance.

- Risk of heart disease in women.
- Risk of prostate cancer in men and ovarian cancer in women.
- Supplementation can slow the production of natural DHEA that your body produces.

Although DHEA is readily available in health food stores and pharmacies without prescription, it is strongly advised only to supplement this hormone under a doctor's supervision. Your doctor will help you determine the dosage you should be taking as well as when it should be taken. Women should be more cautious when supplementing with DHEA as there is a greater risk of negative side effects. It is especially important for women not to supplement with this hormone unless under the care of a physician.

I am currently replacing DHEA in a number of patients. There is no need to replace this hormone unless your levels are low. I have also found it beneficial to supplement DHEA for a few days a week rather than every day as taking too much DHEA can stop your own production of this hormone.

If you are replacing it, take the smallest dose needed to bring this hormone back to the required level and be regularly monitored by your physician.

MELATONIN

Melatonin is secreted by the pineal gland, a small organ located in the brain behind the eyes. Melatonin helps regulate our sleep–wake cycles or circadian rhythms. It is a light sensitive hormone. Levels of melatonin rise rapidly during darkness and fall when we are exposed to light. Even low levels of light can inhibit the production of this hormone. Melatonin levels peak at about age seven and then decline during adolescence. By age 30 the blood levels of melatonin have dropped by 50%.

Not many long–term studies have been done on melatonin, but initial research with humans shows many benefits. Melatonin has been used most often to treat people with sleep disturbances. Sleep deprivation for extended periods of time can lead to stress and a weakening of the immune system. Melatonin has been shown to improve sleep patterns in older people and by so doing, improve their immune function.

Benefits of Replacing Melatonin

- **Induces and improves sleep.** Researchers have been documenting melatonin's sleep inducing properties since the early 1980's when Dr. Richard Wurtzman of MIT's Clinical Research Center started giving volunteers large doses of melatonin. More recent studies have shown that as little as one tenth of a milligram can hasten sleep without the negative side effects of sleeping pills.

- **Melatonin is a powerful antioxidant.** Unlike Vitamin C, which is only active in the aqueous (watery) phase, or Vitamin E, which is only active in the lipid (oily) phase, melatonin is effective in both aqueous and lipid phases.

- **Melatonin shows promise in preventing and treating cancer.** A 1992 study done by Dr. Paolo Lissoni at San Gerardo Hospital in Monza, Italy showed that melatonin significantly increased the one-year survival rates of people with lung cancer. In another study, done by Lissoni on 200 cancer patients with a life expectancy of 6 months, a combination of melatonin and immunotherapy caused the disease to be stabilized in 38% of the patients. Future testing may show that melatonin can play a role in preventing breast and prostate cancers as patients with these diseases have been known to have low melatonin levels.

- **Melatonin is one of the most effective free radical scavengers.** It is most effective in neutralizing hydroxyl radicals, which are responsible for more than half of the free radical damage done to our body. Most other antioxidants become weak free radicals after oxidizing a free radical, but melatonin's antioxidant action involves the donation of two electrons and not one. This ensures that it does not itself become a free radical. Russell Reiter, a University of Texas cellular biologist, has studied melatonin for 30 years and believes melatonin provides more protection against free radicals than any other antioxidant.

- **Improves immune system.** Immune cells are affected by free radicals, thus powerful antioxidants such as melatonin are effective in boosting the immune system.

- **May help establish normal sleep patterns in children with neurological disorders.** Dr. James Jan of Vancouver's British Columbia's Children's Hospital has reported that bedtime doses of between 2.5 to 10 milligrams of melatonin helped establish normal sleep patterns in children with neurological disorders such as epilepsy, Down syndrome, autism and cerebral palsy.

Cautions of Replacing Melatonin

Melatonin should not be taken by:

- Women trying to conceive as high doses can act as a contraceptive
- Nursing mothers or pregnant women as melatonin readily crosses the placenta and studies have not been done on the effect to a developing fetus
- People who have autoimmune diseases such as multiple sclerosis as it can worsen these diseases
- People taking prescription steroid drugs as it can counteract the effectiveness of these drugs
- People with allergies as it can worsen allergic responses
- People treated for depression as it can reduce the effects of some anti-depressant drugs
- Melatonin can reduce the effectiveness of some blood pressure medication

Some studies have shown that melatonin may lessen the symptoms of jet lag and shift work schedules. Several studies done in Britain and France on long distance travelers who change time zones during their flights have shown melatonin reduces the symptoms associated with jet lag by 50%. A more recent study done by the University of Alberta showed no such evidence. Nina Buscemi of the University of Alberta's Department of Pediatrics led a review of 32 melatonin studies involving more than 500 people. The authors of the study wrote in the February 10, 2006 online issue of the *British Medical Journal*, "Our results do not provide evidence that melatonin is effective in alleviating sleep disturbances caused by jet lag."

Although melatonin is available without prescription, it would be wise to consult a physician before replacing this hormone. Some people will be more sensitive to the effects of melatonin. An informed physician will establish the proper dosage required. Melatonin should be taken at bedtime and never during the day. Melatonin does not remain in the bloodstream for very long, therefore taking a time released supplement is more effective. Lower doses are preferred as they seem to have the most beneficial effect on sleep disturbances.

I am currently recommending melatonin to patients who have difficulty sleeping or who travel extensively across time zones. They are taking the lowest dose required to give them a better sleep. Melatonin supplements derived from animals should be avoided.

CHAPTER 7

Growth Hormone

Growth hormone could be the one hormone that may actually reverse the aging process. It is secreted by the pituitary gland and is responsible for:

- promoting growth
- decreasing body fat
- increasing lean muscle tissue
- increasing skin thickness

All of these changes indicate a reversal of the aging process.

Most of this hormone is secreted at night during deep sleep. Secretion of growth hormone decreases as we age, so most people in their 70's have very little in their bloodstream.

The body is still able to make large amounts of growth hormone, but it becomes more difficult to release the hormone from the pituitary gland into the bloodstream. Growth hormone is a short lived hormone in comparison to other hormones. It remains in the bloodstream for only a few minutes. During this time it will target fat cells and the liver stimulating them to release stored fat. This stored fat is used by the body to provide the energy required for building new muscle and for growth.

In 1989, a study was done by Dr. Daniel Rudman and his colleagues at the Medical College of Wisconsin. For a six month period injections of synthetic human growth hormone were given to twelve men whose ages ranged from 61 to 81 years old. All these men lost body fat, increased lean body mass and saw positive improvements in their skin. The conclusion to this study was that growth hormone could reverse the aging process. The men reported changes such as gray hair beginning to go black again, wrinkles disappearing and an increase in energy. Dr. Rudman published these findings in the prestigious *New England Journal of Medicine* on July 5, 1990, writing, "The effects of six months of human growth hormone on lean body mass and adipose–tissue mass were equivalent in magnitude to the changes incurred during 10 to 20 years of aging".

Dr. Rudman did further research on growth hormone administering it to 26 elderly men. He found that their livers and spleens that had shrunken with age had regrown to their youthful sizes.

In 1992, medical researchers at Stanford University arrived at a similar conclusion stating, "It is possible that physiologic growth hormone replacement might reverse or prevent some of the inevitable sequelae of aging."

Following the publication of these reports, many physicians such as Dr. Alan Mintz and Dr. Jeffry Life associated with the Cenegenics Institute in Las Vegas began to replace human growth hormone (HGH) with positive results. In the past 15 years, the use of HGH has increased dramatically in the medical community. The bioidentical synthetic HGH has now been approved by FDA to combat wasting in AIDS patients and for short term use to help patients recover from major surgery or burns.

Studies have indicated that growth hormone not only increases muscle mass, decreases fat and improves skin condition but also has a positive effect on vision, memory, improved wound healing, stronger bones, lower blood pressure, lower LDL cholesterol (bad cholesterol) and improved sexual performance. Kidneys, spleen, heart and liver which normally shrink with age begin to rejuvenate.

When synthetic human growth hormone became available, some athletes began to use this hormone to increase muscle mass, lower fat and improve their performance. They began taking very high doses of growth hormone and this resulted in some unpleasant side effects. Some developed overgrown facial bones, huge hands and feet similar to acromegaly, a genetic disease where the body produces too much growth hormone. As well as excessive bone growth, many grew copious amounts of hair on their entire bodies and others developed carpal tunnel syndrome which led to severe wrist pain. Some studies, including Dr. Rudman's, showed that human growth hormone can cause insulin resistance resulting in the possibility of developing type 2 diabetes.

It is not recommended to supplement with growth hormone if you have enough of your own. When growth hormone is replaced, the body tends to slow down and reduce the normal release of natural hormone. It is best to find a competent physician who is familiar with growth hormone and is willing to have your growth hormone levels tested. If your growth hormone is below the range required for your age, you may consider replacing it.

Most studies showed that small doses have minimal to no side effects. The greatest risks associated with growth hormone such as acromegaly, diabetes and cancer come from using high doses of the hormone. If you do consider replacing growth hormone, then replace only the amount needed to return your growth hormone levels to the normal range.

Benefits of Replacing Growth Hormone

- Decreases body fat
- Increases lean body mass
- Increases skin thickness and reduces wrinkles
- Increases energy
- Tones muscles
- Increases libido
- Increases sense of well-being
- Improves cardiac health
- Improves vascular health

Cautions of Replacing Growth Hormone

- Synthetic growth hormone is normally accepted by the human body, but cases have been reported where the body sees it as a foreign substance and builds anti-bodies to it. There is then a possibility that the immune system will begin to attack its own growth hormone.

- There are natural growth hormones being sold that are made from the pituitary glands of cadavers. These may contain active viruses. Their use was banned in North America after several people developed Creutzfeldt–Jacob disease, also known as mad cow disease.
- There is a possibility of developing type 2 diabetes if excess growth hormone is used.
- There is a possibility of developing carpal tunnel syndrome if excess growth hormone is used.
- There is possibility of experiencing minor joint pain and fluid retention.

I am currently replacing growth hormone in a number of patients. Growth hormone should only be replaced if it is below the required amount for your age. Replace with the smallest dose necessary to bring it back to this level. Replacing growth hormone beyond what is required can cause negative side effects. It is essential to be under a doctor's care and to be monitored frequently if you are replacing this hormone.

CHAPTER 8

Homocysteine

Homocysteine is not a hormone but an amino acid that is found in our bloodstream. It is an important indicator of our health. Homocysteine is created by proteins in our diet that break down to methionine and then to homocysteine. It is necessary for our health as it is associated with the production of several hormones such as dopamine, serotonin, melatonin, adrenaline and also with glutathione which is a detoxifier in our bodies. However, too much homocysteine in the blood can lead to cell damage and major disease such as heart disease and stroke.

The Framingham Heart Study has been doing research on the causes of heart disease for several decades. It was started in 1948 in Framingham, Massachusetts with 5,209 men and women between the ages of 30 and 62 participating in the study. Participants return to the study every two years for detailed medical tests. In 1971, the study enrolled a second generation group of 5,124 participants who were the original participants' adult children and spouses. In April 2002, a third generation, the grandchildren of the original group was included. The first phase of the Third Generation Study with 4,095 participants was completed in July 2005. Over the years, this study has identified some of the major cardiovascular risk factors such as high blood pressure, high blood cholesterol, smoking, obesity, diabetes and physical inactivity.

Framingham investigations indicate that high levels of homocysteine may contribute to heart disease, stroke and reduced flow of blood to the hands and feet. Researchers believe that homocysteine may contribute to the buildup of fatty substances in the arteries, increase the stickiness of platelets and make blood vessels less flexible.

The University of Bergen in Norway is considered to be one of the leading research centers on homocysteine. They have done extensive research and have found that high levels of homocysteine can affect noncardiovascular mortality as well. Work done in 1992 in Hordaland County, Norway with 2,127 men and 2,639 women aged 65 to 67, showed not only an increase in cardiovascular mortality but also an increase in all-cause mortality for people with higher homocysteine levels. High levels of homocysteine can:

- increase risk of heart attack and stroke
- damage arteries
- lead to premature aging
- increase the risk of osteoporosis
- cause damage to the brain and memory
- cause inflammation
- increase risk of certain cancers
- weaken the immune system

In his book called *The H Factor*, Dr. James Braly writes, "Your H score is more important than your weight, your blood pressure or your cholesterol level. It is your most vital, preventable and reversible health statistic." He goes on to say that, "Your homocysteine level is a more accurate predictor than cholesterol of our risk of heart attack or stroke".

Results of studies published in the *New England Journal of Medicine* in May 2004, showed that there is a strong association between homocysteine levels and osteoporosis.

- Research from Holland found that the risk of osteoporosis-related fractures was twice as high in people with homocysteine levels in the top 25% as compared with those with lower levels. A report from Erasmus Medical Center in Holland analyzed data from two studies involving a total of 2,406 people aged 55 or older. Those with the highest levels of homocysteine were 1.9 times more likely than the others to suffer osteoporosis–related fractures.

- A US study involving 825 men and 1,174 women aged 59 to 91 found the risk of osteoporosis–related fractures increased dramatically with homocysteine levels. They were part of the Framingham Heart Study and were followed for 12 to 15 years. Dr. Douglas P. Kiel, the senior author, found men were four times more likely and women two times more likely to have osteoporosis–related fractures when their homocysteine levels were in the top 25% as compared to those in the bottom 25%.

Reducing homocysteine levels will not only decrease your risk for heart disease and osteoporosis, but will improve your immune system, improve your memory and slow the aging process. Men over forty years of age and post-menopausal women are at greater risk of having elevated homocysteine levels.

How Do You Reduce Homocysteine Levels?

- Limit the amount of caffeine
- Eat lean meat and fish
- Eat a clove of garlic daily
- Eat at least 5 servings of vegetables a day
- Limit the amount of salt on foods
- Limit alcohol
- Stop smoking
- Reduce stress and practice a relaxation exercise such as deep breathing or yoga
- Exercise at least 4–5 times a week for 40 minutes
- Take a vitamin and mineral supplement which contains B12, B6, Folic Acid, B2, zinc and magnesium. Folic acid and other B vitamins break down homocysteine in our body.

Testing should be done to determine homocysteine levels as well as B vitamin levels in your bloodstream. If homocysteine is high and folic acid and B vitamins are low, then supplementing your diet with these nutrients would be beneficial. Consult with a physician to determine the supplements you should be taking and the correct dosage of each supplement.

Part II

DIET AND NUTRITION

CHAPTER 9

Diet and Aging

The food we eat influences our hormones, blood glucose, homocysteine and free radical formation, all of which have a major impact on our health and how quickly we age. Keeping our blood chemistry in balance through diet can slow the aging process, as well as ward off disease. Research has shown that diseases, such as type 2 diabetes, heart disease and some cancers can be prevented through proper nutrition.

If we are diagnosed with a medical condition, our doctor might treat the symptoms we have with a variety of drugs rather than finding the underlying problem causing these symptoms. If we are overweight, have high cholesterol, high blood pressure and arthritic pain we could end up with a medication for weight control, another for lowering cholesterol, another for lowering blood pressure, and yet another for arthritis.

All of these drugs are not without consequence. For example, some blood pressure medication works by blocking calcium channels while cholesterol medication and arthritis medication work by manipulating our hormone and enzyme system. We can also experience a negative interaction between the drugs we are given. Diet and lifestyle changes should be tried, before resorting to prescription medication. Proper nutrition alone may be the only medicine we need.

Rather than dispensing drugs for the symptoms that we have, it is imperative to find a physician who is willing to take the time to do the necessary tests and who is knowledgeable in the positive effects that certain foods have.

Many people are intrigued by the new drugs coming on the market and want to try them. We search for a magic potion. Drug companies are gladly willing to assist us with this search. In magazines, on the radio, on bill boards and on television, we are bombarded by drug advertisements. It would appear that there is a special pill for everything, and we are gobbling them up by the handful.

Weight loss diets and diet products are a multibillion dollar industry. In an attempt to lose weight, some people try every diet and pill that is trendy at the time without success.

Why are we failing with these weight loss attempts? Many of the fad diets are so severe that they are impossible to follow. Even worse, many of these diets have a negative impact on our health. They can play havoc with our hormones and blood chemistry and do more harm than good. Often, when we stop one of these trendy diets, we end up gaining even more weight than before.

We have to step back and think about the long term effects that these diets, pills and supplements have on our health. Why do we continue to look for that magic bullet, whether it's a new fad diet or a new and improved diet pill or supplement when all we have to do is fuel our body with the proper nutrition to avoid the problem in the first place? We must change our mindset. We need to get back to the basics of healthy eating and an active lifestyle. We shouldn't look for instant results and search out diets and pills that promise fast weight loss with no regard for our health.

Some people wish to lose weight quickly and restrict calories severely for weeks at a time. They are unable to maintain such a diet long term because they constantly feel hungry. People, who abandon a severe calorie restricted diet and return to their original calorie intake, will begin to gain even more weight than before because their body now burns calories at a slower rate. This may explain why so many people are overweight and why diets fail. Going on and off a severe calorie restricted diet several times a year guarantees a substantial weight gain by the end of the year.

"The Comprehensive Assessment of the Long Term Effects of Reducing Intake of Energy (CALORIE)" study published in the April 5, 2006 issue of the *Journal of the American Medical Association* showed that people on a severe calorie restricted diet had a reduced body temperature. A reduced body temperature slows down the effects of aging, but it also means that the body slows down the rate at which it burns calories.

It is possible to reduce calories, obtain the nutrients we require, feel satiated and maintain a healthy eating plan long term. Being educated on the benefits of certain foods, the negative reaction our body might have to other foods, and how to adjust the portions of the foods we eat to keep calories reduced and hormones balanced will help us make the right choices. Keeping fit and healthy by eating nutritious foods and avoiding foods that disrupt our hormone levels is a lot easier and safer than tormenting ourselves and our body with a variety of weight loss diets and pills.

CHAPTER 10

Metabolic Syndrome

Waistlines in North America and Europe are rapidly expanding. Research predicts that obesity caused by poor diet and lack of exercise will soon surpass tobacco as the leading cause of preventable death. It is estimated that 65 million North Americans suffer from the potentially deadly condition called metabolic syndrome.

Metabolic syndrome puts a person at greater risk for coronary heart disease and diabetes. In 2005 a study was done that indicated that metabolic syndrome also puts a person at risk for chronic kidney disease.

Published in the July 2005 issue of the *American Journal of Nephrology*, the study indicated that people who have metabolic syndrome have an increased long term risk of developing chronic kidney disease. Researchers from the University of California San Francisco followed over 10,000 middle aged Americans in the long-term study of cardiovascular disease risk factors. Originally, none of the subjects had diabetes and all of the subjects had normal kidney function.

In subjects with any of the risk factors of metabolic syndrome, chronic kidney disease was 43% higher than in those with no risk factors. The more risk factors the person had, the higher the likelihood of disease. For subjects that had all the risk factors of metabolic syndrome, the risk was doubled. The results indicate that metabolic syndrome puts middle aged people without diabetes at risk for chronic kidney disease.

Metabolic syndrome is characterized by a group of metabolic risk factors. These include:

- Excessive abdominal fat
- High blood pressure
- Low serum HDL cholesterol and high LDL cholesterol
- High triglycerides
- Insulin resistance
- Elevated blood glucose levels

Metabolic syndrome is defined as having three or more of these risk factors.

The most important risk factors for metabolic syndrome appear to be abdominal obesity and insulin resistance.

It is interesting to note that normal weight people can also have an increased abdominal fat mass and have metabolic syndrome. Waistline measurement will determine if you are carrying too much adipose tissue in the abdominal area.

Abdominal Obesity

A new international study found that waistline measurements can predict cardiovascular disease better than both body mass index and age. More than 170,000 people in 63 countries participated in the "International Day for the Evaluation of Abdominal Obesity (IDEA) Study." A clear relationship between heart disease and the measurement of the waist was found.

- Men who have a waist measurement of 94 centimeters (37 inches) or more and women with a waist measurement of 80 centimeters (31.5 inches) or more are considered abdominally obese and at risk for heart disease. After that, every increase in waist circumference of 14 cm (5.3 inches) for men and 14.9 cm (5.9 inches) for women raises the risk of cardiovascular disease by 19% according to the IDEA study.

Dr. Arya Sharma, director of the Canadian Obesity Network and lead Canadian investigator of the IDEA study, said, "It's not the amount of fat – it is where your fat is located."

Abdominal obesity indicates that there is fat present deep within the abdomen. It is this adipose tissue that increases the risk of developing cardiovascular disease and type 2 diabetes. Adipose tissue is useful for storage and release of energy, but it also produces hormones. Abnormal levels of hormones can cause high blood sugar and high cholesterol levels which can lead to disease.

Insulin Resistance

Excessive insulin is most responsible for accelerated aging. Although insulin is an important hormone for achieving healthy blood sugar levels, too much insulin can cause insulin resistance. Insulin resistance occurs when a person's sensitivity to insulin becomes diminished and they require more and more insulin to maintain blood sugar levels.

If increased amounts of insulin can't keep blood sugar in control, then blood sugar levels climb to above normal readings leading to the development of type 2 diabetes. There has been a huge increase of insulin resistance in North America. Young people in their twenties and thirties are becoming insulin resistant and are developing diabetes.

Insulin resistance has not only been implicated in increasing the risk of developing diabetes but also a wide variety of age related diseases such as high blood pressure, heart disease, stroke and some cancers. A study published in May, 2005 in the journal *Circulation* shows that insulin resistance leads to a shortened lifespan.

The good news is that insulin levels can be controlled by the food we eat.

- To keep the hormones insulin and glucagon in proper balance, protein and low glycemic carbohydrates should be eaten with every meal and snack. Low glycemic carbohydrates are slow–digesting carbohydrates that do not cause a fast increase in blood glucose and insulin when eaten. I will give examples of these later in this chapter.
- To keep insulin and glucagon balanced throughout the entire day, do not skip meals. Three properly balanced meals and two properly balanced snacks should be eaten each day.

Insulin is the hormone responsible for storing incoming nutrients. High levels of insulin will store fat and will also prevent stored fat from being released for use. Carbohydrates and excess calories stimulate insulin to be secreted.

Glucagon is the hormone that sends a message to the body to release stored carbohydrates from the liver and use them to replenish blood sugar levels. When glucagon levels increase, insulin levels decrease. Protein stimulates glucagon to be secreted.

To keep the glucagon/insulin balance in a healthy range, one-third of your meal or snack should be protein and two-thirds should be a low glycemic carbohydrate. For lunch and dinner, an adequate amount of protein would be about the size of your palm. For snacks, the protein size should be cut to approximately one-third of this size.

Make wise food choices. Reduce saturated fats and trans fats. These are linked to a decrease in insulin sensitivity. Select lean meats and poultry and replace whole dairy products with lower fat choices. Other foods that may improve insulin sensitivity are:

■ Whole grain foods have been linked to improved insulin sensitivity. "The Insulin Resistance Atherosclerosis Study", done in the U.S., followed 978 middle-aged participants and found that eating whole grain foods improved insulin sensitivity.

- The mono and polyunsaturated fats that nuts contain may improve insulin sensitivity. The Harvard School of Public Health did a 16 year study on 83,000 women. Participants who ate nuts five times a week or more had a significantly lower risk of developing type 2 diabetes, than those who never or rarely ate them. Nuts, however, have a high fat content and should be eaten in limited amounts. If you are adding more nuts to your diet, eliminate some of the less nutritional saturated fats so as not to gain weight.

- Dark chocolate with at least 70% cocoa has been linked to improved insulin sensitivity. Recent Italian research assessed the effect of dark chocolate on insulin resistance and found improved insulin sensitivity. Researchers at the University of L'Aquilla in Italy found that dark chocolate may decrease blood pressure and allow the body to use insulin more effectively. Again, as with nuts, care must be taken not to overindulge as chocolate is high in fat and calories. Having an ounce of dark chocolate a day could be enough to supply health benefits. If you are adding chocolate to your diet eliminate the less nutritional saturated fats to compensate for the extra calories.

CHAPTER 11

Inflammation

What Is It?

Inflammation is our body's defense against infection and injury. It is the first response of our immune system to infection or injury, and is characterized by redness, swelling, pain and heat. In most cases, inflammation is protective and aids the body in recovery. However, recent studies are showing that chronic inflammation plays a significant role in many diseases, including heart disease, cancer, diabetes, auto-immune diseases and Alzheimer's, and it plays a major role in aging.

Under normal circumstances, inflammation is part of the immune reaction which assists the body in healing. If we cut our finger, white blood cells rush into the injured area to destroy bacteria and repair the torn tissue. The activated white blood cells secrete a number of compounds which promote inflammation. In this case, it is beneficial and helps the body repair the injury. The normal signs of inflammation – heat, soreness, redness and swelling are present for only a short period of time while the wound is healing. This is referred to as acute inflammation.

The harmful kind of inflammation is a low-grade or micro-inflammation that exists undetected for long periods of time. This is referred to as chronic inflammation. There are no symptoms. Individuals can feel completely healthy and are totally unaware that they have this condition.

It was not until the 1990's that medical researchers discovered a link between chronic inflammation and heart disease. The artery walls are not smooth but are a multilayer tissue structure. Researchers found that arteries absorb LDL (bad) cholesterol from the bloodstream, but instead of sticking to the wall of the artery, it actually penetrates into the wall. The imbedded cholesterol becomes inflamed and the combination of cholesterol and inflammation forms an unstable plaque in the artery wall. This area swells, constricting the blood flow to the heart. The artery may be inflamed for a long period of time without the person being aware of it as there are no symptoms. Eventually, the plaque ruptures away from the wall and blocks the artery, which results in heart damage.

Chronic inflammation can cause cells to oxidize and this may trigger formation of many cancer mutations. Bruce Ames, a biochemist at the University of California at Berkeley and former member of the National Cancer Institute, has estimated that inflammation is responsible for up to 30% of all cancers. Cancer patients usually have an elevated level of C-reactive protein (CRP) in their bloodstream. CRP levels are a measure of inflammation; the higher the levels, the more inflammation is present.

Some organs of the body are at greater risk for cancer when they are inflamed. Studies have shown that taking aspirin regularly could reduce the risk of colon cancer. Researchers suspect that the anti-inflammatory drug helps quiet the inflammation which in turn reduces the risk of cancer.

"The Cardiovascular Health Study" showed that people with the highest levels of CRP were three to four times more likely to develop type 2 diabetes than those with the lowest levels of CRP. This again suggests that inflammation plays a role in developing this condition. It may be that diabetes is strongly related to abdominal fat which creates proteins called cytokines that cause inflammation. The more fat cells we have, the more cytokines are present.

Cytokines disrupt insulin production, putting us at risk for type 2 diabetes.

A study was done in Chieti, Italy with obese women who were pear-shaped and carried their fat mainly in their hips and thighs, and obese women who were apple-shaped and carried most of their fat around their abdomen. Results indicated that the women who were apple-shaped were more prone to the low-grade inflammation that can increase the risk of heart disease and stroke. Researchers reported that losing weight would lower their risk, but low-dose aspirin may be considered by some women who fail to lose weight. Aspirin can reduce inflammation in the body. The report was published in the October 30, 2002 issue of the *Journal of the American Medical Association.*

Chronic inflammation is now being implicated in Alzheimer's disease. People who regularly use anti-inflammatory drugs are less at risk of being diagnosed with Alzheimer's disease. It is assumed that the drugs are fighting inflammation, but the mechanism of how they work isn't fully understood. Scientists believe that the drugs may be inhibiting production of the amyloid-beta protein which might be what causes damage to the brain cells of Alzheimer's patients.

There are over 80 different chronic autoimmune diseases that involve almost every human organ system from the gastrointestinal to the blood vessels to the skin. In all these diseases the body's immune system becomes misdirected and begins to attack healthy cells.

Diseases such as multiple sclerosis, rheumatoid arthritis and lupus are known as autoimmune diseases. With these diseases, the body's immune system triggers an inflammatory response even though there is no sign of injury or infection. The normally protective immune system begins to damage healthy cells as if they were in some way infected or a threat.

How is Inflammation Measured?

Inflammation is measured by a marker called C-reactive protein (CRP). The more inflammation that you have in your body, the higher the amount of CRP you will have in your bloodstream. Patients with cancer or autoimmune diseases often have high levels of CRP in their bloodstream. A blood test can determine CRP levels.

This test is making headlines for its ability to detect possible heart disease in people with acceptable cholesterol levels. In a major study published in the *New England Journal of Medicine*, in January 2005, people with elevated CRP levels were four and a half times more likely to have a heart attack.

This makes CRP levels in the bloodstream a valuable predictor of heart disease risk, and may be just as important, or even more important than cholesterol and homocysteine levels.

How Can Inflammation Be Reduced?

Inflammation can be controlled through life-style changes, such as improving your diet, losing weight, exercising, controlling high blood pressure and not smoking.

The foods we eat have a major influence on the amount of inflammation in our bodies. Unlike cholesterol, CRP is not found in food, but diet can greatly affect the levels of this protein in our bloodstream. As blood sugar levels increase, so do CRP levels. Soft drinks, cakes, cookies, refined grains such as white bread and pasta, all raise blood sugar levels quickly, which raises CRP levels. It is best to cut back on, or better still, totally avoid these products.

Losing weight through proper nutrition and exercise is important to control inflammation. Research done by Simin Liu M.D., Ph.D., of the Harvard Medical School, found that a diet high in refined carbohydrates and high glycemic foods (foods that rapidly raise blood sugar levels) increased inflammation. Liu found that women eating large amounts of foods, such as white rice, breakfast cereal, potatoes, white bread and muffins, had elevated CRP levels. Women who were overweight and ate these foods had the highest and most dangerous levels of CRP. Being overweight greatly increases inflammation in the body, as adipose cells, particularly those around the abdomen, make large amounts of CRP.

Dietary fats influence inflammation. Most omega–6 fats, which are found in foods such as margarine, corn oil, peanut oil or soybean oil, tend to cause inflammation. Omega–3 fats, found in fish such as salmon, mackerel or herring and also in flaxseed and leafy green vegetables, have an anti–inflammatory effect on the body. If you don't like eating fish then taking a fish oil supplement may be a good idea.

Vegetables have anti–inflammatory properties. Broccoli, green beans, cauliflower and salad greens contain anti–inflammatory nutrients. These vegetables contain antioxidants which help neutralize free radicals that promote inflammation. They are also rich in alpha–linolenic acid, the basic building block of omega–3 fatty acids.

CHAPTER 12

Weight Loss Diets

Over the past ten years, there has been a rapid increase in obesity and diseases related to poor nutrition. It is interesting to note that over this same time period, many weight loss diets have been introduced. I'm sure all of us are aware of the low fat diet, the low carbohydrate diet and the calorie restricted diet as these were some of the more popular ones.

Low Fat Diets

In the 1990's, research showed that diets that were low in fat and high in fruits, vegetables and grains protected us from disease. As the low fat diet became the new craze, many new products appeared on the shelves that were low in fat or fat free.

Different kinds of snack foods and cookies appeared with "fat free" written on the packages in large letters. We began to eat these instead of fruits and vegetables that are fat free, nutritional, and low in calories. The problem was that many of these fat free foods were not only low in nutrition but also high in calories. These products contained the same number of calories as the original products with normal fat content.

People trying to lose weight began buying and eating these foods, thinking they were making wise choices. Large servings of these snacks were being eaten, without guilt, as they were fat free. More and more people, especially young people, began to gain weight after heavily indulging in fat free foods.

Fat is required in our diet to aid in the control of insulin levels, prevent insulin resistance, and weight gain. Even though fats have no effect on insulin production, certain fats appear to slow down the entry of carbohydrates into the bloodstream. Less insulin is produced if some fat is eaten with the carbohydrate. Not all fats are "good" fats. The best fats to add to your diet are monounsaturated fats, such as those found in olive oil, avocados, nuts and fish. Replace saturated fats in your diet with these more healthy fats.

Low Carbohydrate Diets

We then switched our attention to the low carbohydrate diet. Similar to the low fat craze, different foods began to appear on the shelves with "low carbohydrate" written on the packages. Once again, many people overlooked the benefits of fruits, vegetables and grains and only focused on "low carb" products. Many of these products were low in nutrition and high in calories.

Some people avoided carbohydrates completely and began eating excessive amounts of fat and protein in an attempt to stay slim and healthy. There was a noticeable change in appetite in the people on these diets. At this point, scientists began looking for the reasons behind this change. A study was done that increased the protein content of the subject's diets while keeping the carbohydrates at a constant level of 50%.

The study was published in the *American Journal of Clinical Nutrition* in July 2005. Nineteen subjects were placed on a diet that had:

■ 15% protein, 35% fat and 50% carbohydrate for 2 weeks

Their diet was then adjusted to:

■ 30% protein, 20% fat and 50% carbohydrate for
2 weeks

These regimes contained the same amount of calories and only the fat and protein amounts were varied. The purpose of this part of the study was to determine if the satiety readings would change with the changing amounts of fat and protein.

The results showed that with the first two regimes, the subjects felt fuller on the second regime that had more protein and less fat.

They then went on to the third regime that had the same ratio of protein, fat and carbohydrate as the second regime.

■ 30% protein, 20% fat and 50% carbohydrate for
12 weeks

But this time, the subjects were allowed to eat as much as they wanted to satisfy their appetites; they had no calorie restrictions. The only restriction they had was to maintain the above ratios of protein, fat and carbohydrate.

The results showed that in the third regime the subjects actually ate 450 fewer calories a day. When the subjects ate according to what their appetites dictated, they actually ate fewer calories. They lost more than 10 pounds on average.

People eating protein felt less hungry. It was concluded that adding protein to the diet had the effect of reducing appetite.

Calorie Restricted Diets

Calorie restricted diets have been studied for several decades. In 1935, Clive McCay and Leonard Maynard, two Cornell University food scientists, published the results of a study showing that a low calorie diet is associated with prolonged life. The scientists fed lab rats a diet that was deficient in calories but was adequate in vitamins, minerals, and protein, and compared the results to rats that were fed the same food, but with additional calories. The rats with the lower calorie diet lived longer.

Since this initial work, many studies have been done on various animals with similar findings of increased life span with calorie reduced diets. In 2006, a study to show the effects of calorie restriction was done on humans.

"The Comprehensive Assessment of the Long Term Effects of Reducing Intake of Energy (CALORIE)" study followed 48 participants, eating calorie controlled diets for a six month period. The participants, 27 women and 21 men, were randomly given one of four diets to follow over the test period.

- A diet designed to maintain a constant weight, which was the control group
- A similar diet, but with a 25% reduction of calories
- A similar diet, but with a 12.5% reduction of calories plus enough exercise to increase energy expenditure by another 12.5%
- An extremely low calorie diet designed to quickly drop 15% in body weight and then sufficient calorie intake to maintain the lower weight

After six months, the control group had a measured weight loss of about 1%. The 25% calorie restricted diet and the calorie restricted diet with exercise lost about 10% during the trial. The low calorie diet lost about 14%.

The results of the study were published in the April 5, 2006 issue of the *Journal of American Medical Association* and showed that the participants who ate the calorie reduced diets lost the most weight as expected, but positive results were also observed for the markers of aging.

"Our results show that calorie restriction caused a reversal in two of the three previously reported biomarkers of longevity (fasting insulin and core body temperature)" wrote lead author Leonie Heilbronn, from Louisiana State University.

During the six months of this study, the three groups of participants that ate the low calorie diets showed less damage to their DNA. As people age, their DNA becomes fragmented and damaged. The DNA of the participants who ate the higher calorie diet showed a slow but constant rate of damage, as would be expected. Low calorie diets appear to stave off DNA damage that causes diseases of aging.

However, the problem is that the diet so severely restricts calories that it is unlikely that most people would happily adopt it. Many people don't want to follow such a strict regime for long periods of time. The result of the calorie restricted diet study explains why diets fail and why people gain weight after they stop such a diet.

This study showed that calorie restriction will reduce body temperature and decrease the rate at which we burn calories. If we attempt such a diet, get discouraged and return to a higher calorie diet, we are almost certain to gain even more weight than before, as the rate at which we burn calories has decreased. If we do this several times a year, by the end of the year, we will have gained an excessive amount of weight.

How many times have you heard people lament, "I'm always dieting but seem to gain more weight than I lose?" It is necessary to avoid severe calorie fluctuations, especially when you are trying to lose weight.

Research shows that a calorie restricted diet is beneficial to our health as it slows the effects of aging, lessens the risk of chronic disease, increases lifespan and maintains our weight in a healthy range. It is possible to restrict calories, obtain the nutrients we require and not feel hungry. I will discuss how this can be done.

CHAPTER 13

Developing the Perfect Eating Plan

Many experts believe that to lose weight, one must simply eat fewer calories. However, our body is far more complex than that. It is not only how many calories we eat, but what we eat, and when we eat it that is important.

For example, a bowl of blueberries can have the same amount of calories as a sugar laden cookie, but they will have a very different affect on our body. The cookie, a fast–digesting carbohydrate, will raise blood sugar quickly and signal the body to stop burning fat, forcing the body to use the excess sugar for energy instead. The bowl of blueberries, a slow–digesting carbohydrate, will not raise blood sugar levels as quickly, which allows the body to continue to burn fat. The cookie and the fruit have the same number of calories, but very different effects on your ability to lose body fat.

What we have learned over the years, with the many studies done and weight loss diets tried is that going back to basics may be the most successful way of staying lean.

Balancing Meals

It is essential to balance your meals. If you fill your plate with a slow–digesting carbohydrate, a low fat protein and a healthy fat, you will achieve the most benefit. Every meal and snack should be balanced.

- **Protein is required in every meal or snack.** It reduces appetite and maintains insulin levels in proper balance. With insulin levels in balance, we are less likely to gain weight. Protein stops muscle breakdown and provides the raw materials for producing new muscle.
- **Slow–digesting carbohydrates, such as fruits and vegetables, should be included in every meal, and be the largest portion of the meal.** Slow–digesting carbohydrates replenish energy without causing a rapid increase in blood sugar levels. They

supply most of the vitamins and minerals we require as well as providing us with fiber, which slows digestion and lowers the rate of insulin production. Vegetables contain fewer calories, therefore, we can enjoy large portions of them. When the majority of our plate is fruits and vegetables, we will be consuming fewer calories, will have the benefit of a large supply of nutrients, and will be less likely to feel hungry.

■ **Include a "good" monounsaturated fat with each meal and snack.** Fats play a role in preventing insulin resistance and weight gain. Fat signals the body that more is available permitting it to burn stored reserves.

Frequency of Meals

It is important to eat frequently throughout the day to prevent blood sugar levels from dropping too low. When blood sugar levels drop too low, the body secretes the hormones glucagon and cortisol to return levels back to normal. One of the ways that cortisol increases blood sugar is to convert muscle protein to sugar. Eating frequent meals helps to maintain glucose levels in a healthy range and protects your muscles from being broken down and used for energy.

Small meals throughout the day reduce appetite as well as boost the rate at which calories are burned. It is important not to skip meals, especially breakfast.

If you are overweight, it is particularly important not to skip breakfast. Include some low fat protein such as a scoop of cottage cheese or low fat cheese, an egg, some poultry, fish or lean meat with your breakfast.

- In February 2005, the *American Journal of Clinical Nutrition* reported that skipping breakfast may lead to weight gain as well as increase the risk of heart disease in healthy people over time. The study showed that healthy women who skipped breakfast for two weeks ate more during the rest of the day and developed higher LDL "bad" cholesterol levels than women who ate breakfast every day.
- In a study of almost 2,800 people, Harvard University researchers found that those who ate breakfast every day were 44% less likely to be overweight and 41% less likely to suffer from insulin resistance than those who did not eat breakfast.
- In another study, scientists at the University of Nottingham in the U.K. found that if breakfast was skipped, LDL cholesterol ("bad" cholesterol) readings were elevated, and people were more likely to suffer from insulin resistance.

- A study published in the January 2006 issue of the *Journal of the American College of Nutrition* showed that eating eggs for breakfast instead of a bagel can reduce hunger and caloric intake both at lunchtime and for the next 24 hours. Twenty–eight overweight individuals were randomly assigned an egg–based breakfast or a bagel–based breakfast, both containing the same amount of calories. Researchers found that those that consumed the egg breakfast ate on the average 163 fewer calories at lunch the same day and 418 fewer calories over a 24 hour period of time, than those that ate the bagel breakfast.

Many studies have been done which show that eating several small meals throughout the day has a major benefit to our health.

- The results of a study published in the *British Medical Journal* in December 2001, showed that eating several small meals during the day, as compared to one or two large ones, lowered blood cholesterol in the study participants.

  The study was done in Norfolk, England with 14,666 men and women aged 45 to 75 years and showed that those who ate one or two large meals a day had higher cholesterol levels than those who ate the same calories per day spread over several meals and snacks. Those who ate five or six times a day had the lowest cholesterol readings.

- A study done in 1999 in Johannesburg, South Africa, showed frequent meals reduced appetite by 27%. The results appeared in the *International Journal of Obesity & Related Metabolic Disorders*. Eating smaller meals through-out the day boosts the metabolic rate and the rate at which calories are burned. The subjects eating the frequent meals had more favorable blood glucose and insulin profiles as well.

- Paul Fabry, researcher, came to similar conclusions. He found that if the subjects in his study ate one sixth of their food six times a day, rather than one third of their food three times a day, they had lower cholesterol levels and an improvement in glucose tolerance. Furthermore, they lost weight.

THE PERFECT EATING PLAN

If you incorporate everything I have discussed thus far, you can develop a perfect eating plan specific to you. With the Perfect Eating Plan, you will be enjoying and eating plenty of food, not feeling hungry or deprived, and eating healthier lower calorie meals.

There are three basic requirements:

1. Do not skip meals. Have breakfast, lunch and dinner each day so your body is fuelled throughout the day, your hormones are in balance and you do not feel hungry.

2. Balance each meal with one third of your plate as low fat protein (about the size of the palm of your hand), and two thirds of your plate as slow–digesting carbohydrates such as vegetables, fruits and whole grains. Add to this a small amount of good fat such as nuts, olive oil or avocado, and you will have a meal that will keep your glucose and hormones in balance, and keep you satiated.

3. Have an afternoon snack and an evening snack. Snacks keep your glucose and insulin levels in balance throughout the day and should not be missed. You cannot control your weight unless you control your insulin levels. Each snack should contain a low fat protein, a slow–digesting carbohydrate, and a good fat. For snacks the protein, carbohydrate and fat amount should be cut to about one–third of the meal size.

With this eating plan you will be eating enough food to feel full and satisfied, and you will not be consuming an excessive amount of calories.

If you are overweight when you start this eating plan, you will notice a loss of weight and an increased sense of well-being. The weight you lose will be excess body fat, and it will be permanent if you continue to follow this plan.

It is important not to get discouraged if you are unable to follow your eating plan occasionally. Keep your meals and snacks balanced and if you are unable to do this one day, just go back to balancing your next meal or snack. The Perfect Eating Plan is not a restrictive diet. It is a healthy way of eating. It is a way of balancing meals to keep your glucose and insulin levels in check. This will keep your weight in control and your health at its peak.

Let me now discuss some of the more desirable foods you can choose to create your own Perfect Eating Plan.

CHAPTER 14

Desirable Carbohydrates, Proteins and Fats

When making up your individual eating plans, concentrate on healthy food choices and enjoyable foods.

In 1978, Dr. David Jenkins, a University of Toronto professor, developed a system of ranking foods according to their glycemic index, a calculation that measures how quickly foods are absorbed by our bodies and by how much they raise our blood sugar. The research, done at both the Universities of Toronto in Canada and Oxford in England, was to determine which foods would be best for diabetics.

Individual foods are compared with pure glucose which has its glycemic index set at 100. A slow-digesting carbohydrate would have a low glycemic index under 50. Foods with high glycemic indices are fast-digesting carbohydrates, and these tend to rapidly increase our blood sugar and insulin levels.

- White bread is a fast-digesting carbohydrate and has a high glycemic index. Whole grain bread is a slower digesting carbohydrate and has a lower glycemic index. A one ounce slice of white bread has a glycemic index of 71 and a one ounce slice of whole grain bread has a glycemic index of 51. It is best to select whole grain bread.
- Instant rice has a higher glycemic index than long grain rice. The glycemic index of finely chopped instant oats is higher than large flake, slow-cooking oats. Try to avoid processed foods.
- Overcooking increases the glycemic index of pasta and rice. Select whole grain pasta and wild or brown rice and do not overcook.

Desirable Carbohydrates

These carbohydrates are slower digesting, and have a lower glycemic index:

- Green vegetables (asparagus, green beans, bok choy, artichokes, broccoli, brussels sprouts, cabbage, leeks, spinach, swiss chard, kale, snow peas, celery)
- Eggplant
- Zucchini
- Cauliflower
- Squash
- Turnip
- Bell peppers (red, yellow, green)
- Mushrooms
- Radishes
- Onions
- Tomatoes
- Sauerkraut
- Turnip
- Garlic
- Apples
- Citrus fruit (oranges, grapefruit)
- Berries (strawberries, blueberries, blackberries, boysenberries, cherries)
- Kiwis
- Grapes
- Peaches
- Pears
- Plums

Beans and Legumes

- Kidney beans
- Chickpeas
- Black beans
- Lentils
- Dried peas

Grains

- Whole grain breads
- Brown rice
- Slow cooking oatmeal
- Barley

Desirable Protein

- Fish (bass, cod, haddock, salmon, mackerel, sardines, snapper, trout, tuna)
- Scallops
- Shrimp
- Lobster
- Turkey breast, skinless

- Turkey bacon
- Ground turkey
- Lean beef
- Lean pork
- Chicken breast, skinless
- Low fat milk
- Low fat cheese
- Plain, low fat yogurt
- Eggs and egg whites
- Tofu
- Vegetarian protein, such as soybean bacon, sausage, hamburger or hot dog

Desirable Fats

- Olive oil
- Canola oil
- Fish oils
- Nuts
- Avocados
- Sunflower seeds
- Flaxseeds

HEALTHY FOOD CHOICES

We should concentrate on only healthy food choices. If we fill our plates with healthy foods, it leaves little room for the less wholesome foods. I will now discuss some of the recent studies done describing the health benefits of a few of these food choices.

Fruits and Vegetables

One benefit to eating plenty of fruits and vegetables is that these foods are low in calories. We can eat more of them and are less likely to feel hungry after a meal. Filling our plate with slow-digesting carbohydrates, such as fruits and vegetables, not only curbs the amount of calories we eat, but also satisfies our appetite. This diet provides many other benefits as well.

A study, published in the January 10, 2006 issue of *Journal of the American College of Cardiology*, found that a diet rich in fruits and vegetables benefits the heart. The study looked at the heart function of 25 subjects aged 41 to 64, who consumed 1,400 to 2,000 nutritionally balanced calories per day.

The subjects ate a diet similar to the Mediterranean diet, with plenty of fruits and vegetables, beans, whole grains, olive oil and fish. They avoided refined and processed foods, soft drinks, desserts, white bread and other fast–digesting carbohydrates. They were compared to 25 people who ate a typical Western diet, consuming 2,000 to 3,000 calories per day.

The results showed that the people on the more nutritious and calorie reduced diet had the heart function of a person 15 years younger than their age. The study also suggested that eating this nutritious diet, loaded with vegetables, can also reduce the risk of cancer.

Lead author of the study, Luigi Fontana, assistant professor of medicine at Washington University in St. Louis, said, "This is the first study to demonstrate that long–term calorie restriction with optimal nutrition has cardiac–specific effects that (delay or reverse) age–associated declines in heart function."

Most people abandon calorie restricted diets because while on these diets they always feel hungry. Fruits and vegetables are filling and supply a cornucopia of nutritional benefits without being high in calories. Consequently, you are eating lower calorie meals, are not hungry and are more likely to maintain a calorie reduced eating plan.

Every fruit and vegetable offers a different array of nutrients. In order to get the full range of nutrients, it is wise to consume a wide assortment of fruits and vegetables, and not continually eat just one or two favorites. Even different varieties of the same fruit can have different nutrients. For example, different varieties of apples supply different antioxidants.

- **Apples** supply antioxidants known as flavonoids, which have been linked to providing protection against heart disease. Eat different varieties of apples to benefit from different antioxidants.
- **Tomatoes** supply lycopene which may provide protection against prostate cancer. If the tomatoes are cooked, the amount of lycopene that is absorbed substantially increases. Eat tomatoes both cooked and raw. If the tomatoes are raw, the gel found around the seeds may have anti–blood clotting action which may provide heart health benefits.
- **Citrus fruits** provide phytochemicals, flavonoids, folate, postassium, vitamin C, fiber, and limonoids, which have been associated with providing protection against certain cancers. Different citrus fruits provide different phytochemicals. It is beneficial to eat a variety of citrus fruits and not always choose the same fruit.
- **Cranberries** decrease the risk of certain infections because of their bacterial anti–adhering properties.

- **Broccoli and cauliflower** may provide protection against cancer. A report published in the January 5, 2000 issue of the *Journal of the National Cancer Institute*, showed men who ate 28 or more servings of vegetables per week had a 35% lower risk of prostate cancer compared to those who ate fewer than 14 servings per week. Additionally men who ate three or more servings of cruciferous vegetables per week, such as broccoli and cauliflower, had a 41% less risk of prostate cancer compared to those that ate one serving or less per week. The study was done on 648 participants aged 40 to 64 who had been newly diagnosed with prostate cancer as well as 604 cancer–free men of the same age. The researchers theorized that cruciferous vegetables are high in isothiocyanates, which activate enzymes that detoxify carcinogens.

- **Mushrooms** have been shown to improve the function of the immune system. Researchers from Penn State University have found that mushrooms, such as shitake, oyster, maitake and portabellas, contain high levels of the antioxidant, ergothioneine that is associated with protection against chronic disease.

- **Onions** contain flavonoids, which may provide protection against heart disease and cancer. Onions retain flavonoids even after they are cooked.

- **Hot peppers** may defend against prostate cancer. Research done by Cedars–Sinai Medical Center at the University of California at Los Angeles found that capsaicin, the pungent ingredient in hot peppers, causes prostate cancer cells to self–destruct. The researchers reported that these results show that capsaicin may have a role in the management of prostate cancer patients, even for those men who don't respond to hormone therapy.

Blueberries

Blueberries are loaded with antioxidants, anthocyanocides, bacterial inhibiters, folic acid, carotenoids, vitamins A and C, and dietary fibers which help fend off disease.

- Researchers at the USDA (U.S. Department of Agriculture) Human Nutrition Center rated blueberries first in antioxidant activity when compared to 40 other fruits and vegetables. Antioxidants help neutralize free radicals that can lead to cancer and other age-related diseases.
- Studies done at the University of California at Davis showed that blueberries may reduce the build up of

"bad" cholesterol that contributes to heart disease and stroke. Antioxidants are believed to be responsible for this health benefit.

- Researchers at Rutgers University in New Jersey have identified a compound in blueberries that promotes urinary tract health and reduces the risk of infection by preventing bacteria from adhering to the walls of the urinary tract.

- European and Japanese studies indicate that antho-cyanin, the blue pigment in blueberries, may have a positive effect on eyesight and may ease eye fatigue.

- A USDA Human Nutrition Center study showed that blueberries may slow age-related loss in mental capacity and may keep Alzheimer's disease at bay. James Joseph, Ph.D., and his team showed that a diet of blueberries may improve motor skills and reverse the short-term memory loss that comes with aging and age-related diseases, such as Alzheimer's.

- A study published in the *Journal of Nutritional Biochemistry*, February 2006, showed that blueberries may strengthen blood vessels and protect them against oxidative stress and inflammation that can lead to heart disease.

- A study published in the *Journal of Food Science* in 2005 and conducted by Mary Ann Lila, Ph.D., at the University of Illinois, indicates that compounds in wild blueberries may be effective inhibitors of cancer. The findings conclude that wild blueberry compounds have the potential to attack all stages of cancer – initiation, promotion and proliferation. According to the study, different types of wild blueberry compounds are active during different stages of cancer. This results in a broad spectrum of potential cancer fighting benefits.

Cranberries

About 20 years ago, scientists at Youngstown State University found that cranberry juice inhibited E. coli bacteria, the bacteria most responsible for urinary tract infections, from adhering to the urinary tract.

Testing done by scientists at Rutgers University has showed that cranberries have compounds called proantho-cyanidins that they believe are responsible for the microbial anti-adhesion property. Although grape and apple juices also have these compounds, their proanthocyanidins do not appear to have this unique feature.

Professor Amy B. Howell, a researcher at Rutgers University, found that consuming cranberries twice a day is more beneficial than having them only once a day. The non-adhesion effect begins within two hours of consumption of cranberries, but lasts only for about 10 hours, therefore getting a dose of cranberries in the morning and again in the evening is the best way to maintain these anti-adhesion properties.

- A total daily serving of eight to ten ounces of cranberry juice, one and one half ounces of dried cranberries or half a cup of cranberry sauce provides the required dose of proanthocyanidins. Consuming cranberries regularly can decrease the incidence of urinary track infections by 40%.

The same anti-adhesion effects have been demonstrated on other bacteria such as H. pylori. This bacterium is known to be a major cause of stomach ulcers and is suspected to increase the risk of stomach cancer.

Researchers are currently looking at cranberries and tooth decay. The bacterium that causes tooth decay adheres to the surface of the teeth causing plaque to form, and eventually, the teeth to decay. Cranberries could have the same anti-adhesion effect on this bacterium.

Additionally, cranberries, like other berries, are loaded with antioxidants and may offer protection against some cancers as well as provide heart health benefits.

Garlic

For years, allium vegetables such as garlic, chives, onions, leeks and scallions, have been used for medicinal purposes. In 1858, Louis Pasteur demonstrated garlic's anti-bacterial properties. During the First World War, garlic was used to stop the spread of gangrene.

Scientific information was presented in the Washington, D.C. symposium called "Significance of Garlic and Its Constituents in Cancer and Cardiovascular Disease". The proceedings were published in a supplement to the *Journal of Nutrition*. Findings indicate that garlic appears to have many benefits and it may:

- Inhibit the production of cholesterol.
- Decrease the rate of cholesterol oxidation. Oxidized cholesterol is thought to be a likely cause of artery damage.
- Protect against inflammation and damage to the small blood vessels. This damage is associated with Alzheimer's disease and a decrease in cognitive function.
- Protect against stomach, colon, breast, prostate, lung and liver tumors. Animal research shows that garlic can stop the spread of cancer cells and in some cases actually kill cancer cells.

■ Maintain a healthy immune system.

■ Reduce blood pressure.

■ Lower risk of heart attack and stroke because garlic is linked to a slower rate of blood clotting.

Garlic has a complex chemistry with a number of compounds that may work individually or together to produce the health benefits. For this reason, it is best to eat garlic rather than to take garlic supplements. For example, garlic contains:

■ Compounds such as allicin and allyl–thiosulfinate, which may destroy H. pylori bacteria, one of the causes of stomach ulcers. The compound allicin may also protect the heart.

■ The compound diallyl sulfide, which may have anti–cancer properties.

■ The nutrient selenium, which may have anti–cancer properties.

The same health benefits might not be obtained with garlic supplements as they may not have all the compounds that garlic has. Also, the combination of the compounds found in garlic may be more effective when they are in their natural concentrations.

ConsumerLabs.com is a group that tests the quality of supplements. They have found that there is a wide variation in the amount of active ingredients in garlic supplements. Some supplements may not have enough of a certain ingredient, such as allicin, to be effective; others may have too much, and this could interfere with prescribed medication.

Effectiveness of fresh garlic is dependant on how quickly garlic is cooked after crushing. A study done by Maryland scientists showed that garlic's effect on breast cancer tumors is lessened if the garlic is crushed and cooked immediately. When the crushed garlic was allowed to stand for 10 minutes before it was cooked, then it retained more of the cancer fighting ingredients.

Beans and Legumes

Beans, dried peas, lentils and chickpeas are all linked to decreasing the risk of heart disease, stroke, diabetes, obesity and certain cancers. They are loaded with protein, B vitamins, folate, calcium, magnesium, potassium, phosphorus, zinc, copper, iron and both soluble and insoluble fiber.

High levels of non–digestible fibers have been shown to raise HDL "good" cholesterol levels as well as provide better blood sugar regulation. The fiber and the starches in beans and legumes lead to a slower rate of digestion and a more gradual rise in blood sugar levels. This can help in preventing diabetes and controlling sugar levels in those that already have diabetes. Beans and legumes:

- May reduce the risk of obesity. Fiber is linked with a greater sense of satiety. The bulking effect of the fiber in the stomach promotes the feeling of fullness for a longer period of time. The recommended fiber intake per day should be 25 to 30 grams. A half cup serving of chickpeas provides more than six grams of fiber, which is almost one-quarter of the required daily intake.

- Contain isoflavones in varying amounts, which have been found to reduce the risk of heart attack and stroke. Isoflavones decrease the rate of blood clotting. They also act as antioxidants inhibiting formation of oxidized LDL cholesterol, the cholesterol most likely to be deposited in the arteries. Chickpeas have the highest levels of isoflavones.

- Contain phytosterols which have been shown to reduce the risk of certain cancers. A study done by the State University of New York at Buffalo, New York and published in the December 2001 issue of *European Journal of Cancer Prevention* compared the differences between Asian diets rich in phytosterols and Western diets rich in cholesterol. The phytosterol diet appeared to reduce prostate tumor growth by more than 40% and cut the occurrence of cancer spread to other parts of the body by almost 50%. Other research is pointing to protection by phytosterols against colon and breast cancers as well.

Keep cans of chickpeas or beans in the cupboard to make nutritious dips and spreads. Blend these in a food processor with garlic, olive oil, parsley, tahini or cumin and serve with whole grain crackers or pita to create healthy snacks. Beans and lentils can be added to soups and salads. Kidney beans or chickpeas can be added to vegetable soups or can be mixed with red onion, tomatoes, tuna or chicken and tossed with an olive oil and vinegar dressing for a nutritious meal.

When using canned products, drain them and rinse them several times with water in order to reduce the sodium content.

Dark Chocolate

This section is unusually long. I really like eating chocolate!

In recent years, many studies have been done on dark chocolate which show that it has positive benefits to our health. Researchers at the University of L'Aquilla in Italy found that dark chocolate may decrease blood pressure and allow the body to use insulin more effectively. They reported in *Hypertension: Journal of the American Heart Association* that a 100 gram daily serving of flavonoid rich dark chocolate can have a positive effect on blood pressure, insulin and LDL (bad) cholesterol.

Jeffrey B. Blumberg, Ph.D., the study author said, "Previous studies suggest flavanoid–rich foods, including fruits, vegetables, tea, red wine, and chocolate, might offer cardiovascular benefits, but this is one of the first clinical trials to look specifically at dark chocolate's effect on lowering blood pressure among people with hypertension." Blumberg is a senior scientist at the Jean Mayer USDA Human Nutrition Research Center on Aging at Tufts University in Boston.

Ten men and ten women participated in the study. All of them had mild hypertension with systolic blood pressure between 140 and 159 millimeters of mercury and diastolic pressure between 90 and 99 millimeters of mercury. None of the participants took antihypertensive drugs or smoked. During the study, half of the people ate 100 grams of dark chocolate, and the other half ate the same amount of white chocolate. After avoiding flavanoid rich foods for a week, the participants switched over and ate the opposite type of chocolate.

Researchers found a 12 millimeters of mercury decrease in systolic pressure and a 9 millimeters of mercury decrease in diastolic pressure after 15 days, in the group that ate dark chocolate. The blood pressure of the people consuming the white chocolate did not change. The dark chocolate group also had a reduction in insulin resistance as well as a drop in LDL (bad) cholesterol.

"This is not only a statistically significant effect, but it is also a clinically meaningful decline", Blumberg said. "This is the kind of reduction in blood pressure often found in other healthful dietary interventions."

The health benefits of dark chocolate are attributed to the fact that it contains high levels of flavonoids which are powerful antioxidants. Flavonoids have been shown to inhibit blood clot formation, help blood vessels relax and slow the oxidation of LDL cholesterol. It is thought that flavonoids trigger the release of compounds that increase blood flow in the arteries.

Flavonoids are not only found in chocolate, but can be found in nuts, fruits, vegetables and herbs. Thousands of flavonoids exist such as quercetin in apples and onions, polyphenols in berries and red wine, and catechins in black and green tea and dark chocolate. Dark chocolate appears to contain more flavonoids than any other food. Dark chocolate contains about five times as much antioxidant activity as do blueberries.

Researchers from Finland found that among 10,000 men and women, those with the highest flavonoid intake had a 46% lower risk of developing lung cancer and a lower risk of dying from heart disease.

Although dark chocolate contains flavonoids, it also contains fat and calories; 100 grams of dark chocolate would have about 30 grams of fat from cocoa butter and about 500 calories. It is important not to overindulge and if you're adding chocolate to your diet, cut back on other fats or exercise more in order not to gain weight.

A recent study indicates that only 10 grams of dark chocolate a day may be all that is needed to see positive benefits in blood pressure and reduce the risk of dying from heart disease and stroke. The study appeared in the journal *Archives of Internal Medicine* in February 2006 and showed that men with a cocoa consumption equal to that of 10 grams a day were half as likely as others to die from cardiovascular disease.

Researchers from the Centre of Nutrition and Health in Bilthoven, the Netherlands, tracked 470 men, aged 65 to 84, and found that men with the highest cocoa consumption were less likely to die of any cause, not only cardiovascular disease. The study suggests that cocoa may help prevent premature death. It may be that there is an accumulative benefit over time, and that long-term consumption of smaller amounts of chocolate could be just as beneficial.

To get the most benefit from dark chocolate it should have at least 70% but preferably 85% or more cocoa solids. Milk chocolate is about 40% solids at most. Dark chocolate that has flavors such as orange or raspberry added or dark chocolate with caramel or crisps added tends to have more sugar and less flavonoids.

It is very easy to get excited about the benefits of eating a treat as tasty as chocolate. It is fine to indulge in a piece of dark chocolate, but we should keep in mind that fruits and vegetables not only have flavonoids but also have other beneficial nutrients and fewer calories. We should not eliminate these from our diet in exchange for chocolate.

Nuts

Nuts and seeds are a rich source of antioxidants and other compounds with anti-cancer action. Sesamol, found in sesame seeds, has been shown to suppress cancer growth, and melatonin, found in walnuts, may play a role in decreasing breast cancer risk. Nuts and seeds contain several types of vitamin E, such as alpha–tocopherol, gamma–tocopherol and delta–tocopherol. These offer more health benefits than a vitamin E supplement containing only alpha–tocopherol.

Decreasing the amount of saturated and trans fats, and increasing healthy fats, such as those found in nuts, seeds, fatty fish and olive oil will decrease the risk of disease. The fats in these foods have been found to lower the levels of LDL "bad" cholesterol, and increase the levels of HDL "good" cholesterol. An Australian study found that eating 30 grams of walnuts daily, significantly increased the readings of HDL cholesterol, and lowered the readings of LDL cholesterol in people with type 2 diabetes. Research at Loma Linda University in 1993 demonstrated that a diet containing walnuts reduced blood levels of LDL cholesterol and heart disease risk more effectively than the low fat diet recommended by the American Heart Association.

Nuts may play a role in weight control. The *International Journal of Obesity* published a study done by scientists at Purdue University which showed that participants who snacked on peanuts or peanut butter were not hungry again for about two and a half hours. If they snacked on high–carbohydrate snacks, such as rice cakes, they were hungry again within 30 minutes. Even though the peanuts and peanut butter were high in calories, the participants adjusted their caloric intake spontaneously, and did not add extra calories to their diets.

Eating large amounts of nuts throughout the day will certainly cause a weight gain, but having an ounce of nuts a day can provide a number of health benefits. Nuts are a good source of protein, fiber and good fat. They play a role in controlling blood sugar and appetite.

It is wise to substitute the less desirable fat, such as saturated or trans fat with the more desirable fat found in nuts. If you replace saturated and trans fat with the fat found in nuts, you won't notice a weight increase and you will profit from the many health benefits they offer. It may be best to set aside a portion of nuts in the morning, and then have them with meals or as a healthy snack during the day. That way you won't be tempted to overindulge and gain weight.

Whole Grain

Whole grain refers to the entire kernel of the grain – the bran, the germ and the endosperm. Whole grains are rich in vitamins, minerals, lignans, phytosterols and fiber. They are associated with reduced risk of disease. Refined products have the nutrient rich bran and germ removed during the refining process. They lack the fiber and the range of nutrients and disease fighting compounds or phytochemicals.

A study, done with 500 subjects aged 60 to 98, found that those subjects that consumed the most whole grains were half as likely to have metabolic syndrome as those who consumed less than one serving of whole grains per day. They were also half as likely to die from cardiovascular disease in the next decade. In addition, individuals eating the most whole grains weighed less and had lower blood sugar levels. The study was published in the January 2006 issue of the *American Journal of Clinical Nutrition.*

Whole grains may lower cholesterol, decrease the formation of blood clots that can lead to heart attack and stroke, improve the regulation of blood sugar and have a positive effect on the lining of the artery walls.

Some studies have indicated that whole grains may contain substances that increase the rate at which we burn calories. A study published in the *American Journal of Clinical Nutrition* in December 2004, tracked more than 27,000 men over an eight year period, and found that those who consumed the most whole grains gained the least amount of weight.

The most benefit is shown with three servings a day. In 2005, U.S. Dietary Guidelines recommended that at least three one ounce equivalents of whole grain be consumed per day for each adult. A study done with 2,800 subjects, by the Human Nutrition Research Center on Aging at Tufts University in Boston, showed that eating three servings a day of whole grains can play a role in preventing the development of metabolic syndrome. Whole grains are linked to better regulation of blood sugar and better functioning of insulin.

A study published in the July 2005 issue of the *American Heart Journal*, showed that whole grains can offer benefit to those who already have heart disease. Women with a history of heart disease who ate six or more servings of whole grains per week had a slower rate of narrowing of arteries over a three year period.

Whole grains are a source of antioxidants which may play a role in reducing cholesterol deposits in the artery walls. They also contain potassium and magnesium, nutrients which may reduce the risk of developing high blood pressure.

When looking for whole grain products, read the label. The label should read 100% whole grain. Enriched wheat or 100% wheat is refined and not 100% whole grain. Products that are labeled multigrain, oats, rye, 12–grain, etc. can be mostly refined grain. You can't judge bread by color either. Coloring agents, such as caramel, may be added to give the food a dark color. Read the label to ensure you are buying a whole grain product.

In order to meet your quota of three servings a day, add a one half cup of whole wheat pasta or a one half cup of brown rice to your meals. Barley not only contains cholesterol lowering fiber, but also a phytochemical that decreases cholesterol production. Many whole grains are now available, such as quinoa, kamut, splet, millet, sorghum and amaranth. Substitute these for refined grains, such as white rice.

Many people shy away from the less common grains with unusual names, such as quinoa. This small, round, grain comes from a plant in the Andes. Quinoa is an excellent source of protein as one cup contains about 11 grams. It is also rich in fiber, B vitamins, iron, calcium, magnesium and zinc. It's a nutritional powerhouse. It cooks quicker than most grains, has a delicious flavor and a low glycemic index.

Oatmeal is one of the richest sources of soluble fiber. It can lower cholesterol, regulate blood sugar levels and lower the risk of gallstones.

A study published in the December 1996 issue of *Circulation* followed 22,000 Finnish men and found that "an increase in daily soluble fiber intake by three grams reduced the risk of coronary death by 27%". Researchers believe that soluble fiber may also decrease the levels of blood glucose, insulin, triglycerides and fats found in the blood directly after a meal. Research has suggested that a three gram increase in daily soluble fiber, which is about one and a half cups of cooked oatmeal, would benefit heart health.

A study published in the December 1996 issue of *The American Journal of Clinical Nutrition* showed that diets high in oat soluble fiber lowered triglyceride levels. Elevated triglyceride levels are a risk factor for heart disease.

Olive Oil

Olive oil contains a high content of monounsaturated fatty acids as well as a high content of antioxidants that provide protection against disease.

Studies have shown that olive oil offers protection against heart disease by raising the HDL or "good" cholesterol levels while lowering the LDL or "bad" cholesterol levels. Subjects, who consumed about two tablespoons of virgin olive oil a day for a week, showed less oxidation of LDL cholesterol and more antioxidants in their blood.

Extra virgin olive oil, from the first pressing of olives and extracted without using heat or chemicals, is less processed and contains higher levels of antioxidants, particularly vitamin E and phenols.

A study, in the March 27, 2000 issue of *Archives of Internal Medicine*, showed that olive oil may reduce blood pressure. People on high blood pressure medication may be able to reduce the amount of medication they take if they substitute olive oil for other types of fat in their diet. During a 12 month study, subjects who consumed extra virgin olive oil required 48% less antihypertensive medication, while subjects who consumed sunflower oil required 4% less antihypertensive medication. The polyphenol content in olive oil may be one reason for the reduction in blood pressure. Polyphenols are potent antioxidants which help arteries dilate, thereby reducing blood pressure.

"The most important finding in this study is that daily use of olive oil, about 40 grams a day, markedly reduces the dosage of (blood pressure medication) by about 50% in patients on a previously stable drug dosage" says L. Aldo Ferrara, M.D., Associate Professor of Internal Medicine at the Frederico II University of Naples in Naples, Italy, and the study's author.

Another study, done at the University of Oxford, showed that olive oil is as effective as fruits and vegetables in keeping colon cancer at bay. Dr. Michael Goldacre and a team of researchers at the Institute of Health Sciences compared cancer rates, diets and olive oil consumption in 28 mostly European countries but also other countries such as Canada, the United States, Brazil, Colombia and China. The September 2000 study was published in the *Journal of Epidemiology and Community Health*, Goldacre said, "Olive oil may have a protective effect on the development of colon cancer." Researchers suspect that olive oil cuts the amount of deoxycyclic acid and regulates the enzyme diamine oxidase which may be linked to cell division in the bowel.

Olive oil contains flavonoids, squalene and polyphenols which may protect against breast and skin cancer. Flavonoids and polyphenols are antioxidants, which protect cells from damage by free radicals.

Researchers reporting in the September 1, 2005 issue of the journal *Nature* have shown that fresh extra virgin olive oil contains a natural compound, oleocanthal, which is a non-steroidal anti-inflammatory agent that has the same pain relieving activity as drugs, such as ibuprofen.

Paul Breslin, a scientist with the Monell Chemical Senses Center in Philadelphia, who was one of the scientists that directed the research said, "The Mediterranean diet, of which olive oil is a central component, has been long associated with numerous benefits including decreased risk of stroke, heart disease, breast cancer, lung cancer, and some dementias. Similar benefits are associated with some NSAIDs, such as aspirin and ibuprofen. Now we know of oleocanthal's anti-inflammatory properties, it seems plausible that oleocanthal plays a casual role in the health benefits associated with diets where olive oil is the principal source of fat."

Not all olive oils contain oleocanthal. Breslin says the easiest way to determine if an olive oil contains oleocanthal is to taste it. It contains oleocanthal if it triggers a throat sting or an irritation at the back of the throat. Tuscany olive oils usually contain high levels of oleocanthal, which are destroyed by aging and cooking.

Fish

Fish is an excellent protein choice as it has a high content of healthy unsaturated fats. Fish, particularly fatty fish such as salmon, lake trout, sardines, mackerel and herring are a good source of omega-3 fatty acids. Omega-3 fatty acids protect the heart against disease. They decrease triglyceride levels, decrease the rate of artherosclerotic plaque formation, decrease risk of arryhythmias and lower blood pressure.

Numerous studies have recently been published on the many benefits of eating fish. A study published in the November 2006 issue of Archives of Neurology showed that eating fish three times a week may cut the risk of dementia by almost 50%.

Another study done in June 2005 at Indiana University in Bloomington found omega-3 fatty acids may benefit people with exercise-induced asthma. Subjects taking 5.2 grams of omega-3 daily for three weeks saw a 64% improvement in breathing.

Exercise-induced asthma triggers a narrowing of the airways and coughing and wheezing after vigorous exercise. It discourages people from participating in sports and other physical activities as well as hinders competitive athletes. Asthma medication can be affective, but it may have side effects and some medications are banned in international competitions.

A study at Harvard found that the more fish expectant mothers ate during their second trimesters, the better their infants did on tests taken when they were six months old. The study conducted by Emily Oken and colleagues at the Harvard Medical School in Boston, involved 135 mothers and babies. Researchers found that eating fish during pregnancy was positively associated with enhanced fetal brain development and that the more fish the mother ate, the better her six month old scored on standard mental tests.

However, infants whose mothers ate fish that contained high levels of mercury did not see the same boost in mental test scores. The scores of these babies went down as the mercury level went up. Pregnant mothers are advised to avoid large and long-lived fish, such as shark, swordfish, king mackerel, and tilefish, which tend to have higher mercury levels. The study was reported in the October 2005 issue of *Environmental Health Perspectives*.

A study published in *Surgical Neurology* shows that omega-3 fatty acids may reduce and/or prevent inflammation. The mechanism of the anti-inflammatory action involves the conversion of the fatty acids into the anti-inflammatory prostaglandins (PGs) of the PGE 3 series. In the study, researchers supplemented the diets of 125 people with non-surgical spine pain, and who were taking non-steroidal anti-inflammatory drugs (NSAID). The subjects were given daily supplements of 2,400 milligrams of omega-3 fatty acids for two weeks and then 1,200 milligrams per day thereafter. The supplements contained 200 milligrams of DHA, 850 milligrams of EPA and 180 milligrams of other omega-3 fatty acids.

After 2 weeks the participants were asked to stop taking their NSAID medication and after one month they were asked about joint and spine pain and side effects. Sixty per cent said that their overall level of pain had improved since starting the supplements. Fifty-nine per cent said that they had stopped the NSAID medication completely.

The researchers reported, "Eighty per cent of the respondents stated they were satisfied with their improvement and eighty-eight per cent stated they would continue to take the omega-3 essential fatty acids".

The positive preliminary result, and the lack of side effects, led the researchers to propose that as many as two-thirds of people currently taking NSAID medication could discontinue use and benefit from omega-3 fatty acids to alleviate pain from inflammation.

If you wish to take supplements it is best to choose a pharmaceutical grade of fish oil that is free of contaminants, such as heavy metals, mercury, PCBs and dioxins.

Beverages

The World Health Organization recommends that not more than 10% of our calorie intake should come from beverages. Currently, North Americans consume about 21% of their calories from beverages.

Many people are unaware of the amount of calories they consume when drinking beverages, such as chai latte, cola, double-double coffee, iced cappuccino, beer and alcohol. A frozen margarita has the same number of calories as a piece of pizza.

The Beverage Guidance Panel was started by a group of nutrition experts from institutions like Johns Hopkins and Harvard universities to provide guidance on the health and nutritional benefits and risks of various beverage categories. Their goal was to help people understand how to choose healthy beverages as part of a balanced diet.

They reviewed the scientific research on a number of beverage categories, such as water, milk, juices, alcohol and soft drinks. They then ranked the beverages based on calorie intake, nutritional value, and for beneficial and adverse health effects. The beverages were ranked in six levels, level one being the best beverage choice and level six being the worst.

- **Level 1 is water.** Water is without calories and is considered the best beverage. It is necessary for metabolism and for normal physiological functions. Water is essential for our health. Dehydration decreases alertness, concentration and short–term memory.
- **Level 2 is tea and coffee.** Tea provides a variety of flavonoids and antioxidants which can provide protection against disease. Drinking tea and coffee has been linked to many health benefits. Several studies observed there is a decrease in the risk of colon cancer, liver cancer, type 2 diabetes and Parkinson's disease in coffee drinkers.
- **Level 3 is low fat or skim milk and soy beverages.** Milk is a good source of calcium and vitamin D as well as high quality protein. Fortified soymilk is a good alternative for those who do not wish to drink cows' milk.

- **Level 4 is non–calorically sweetened beverages such as "diet drinks".** These beverages provide water and sweetness, without the calories, thus are preferred to calorie loaded drinks.

- **Level 5 is caloric beverages with some nutrients, such as fruit juices and alcohol.** Fruit juices provide some nutrients, but they don't contain the fiber and some of the phytochemicals that a whole fruit would have. They are less filling than the actual fruit, and have higher calories. Moderate consumption of alcohol in adults has shown to have some health benefits, but alcoholic beverages contain calories. Women should have no more than one drink per day, and men no more than two.

- **Level 6 is the calorically sweetened beverages, such as soft drinks.** These are the least recommended beverages. Sweetened soft drinks contain high fructose corn syrup or sucrose, and are linked to weight gain, type 2 diabetes and dental problems. Because of the huge quantities of these beverages consumed, and the high number of calories they contain, soda drinks and fruit drinks most likely contribute to the obesity epidemic.

Healthy Beverage Choices

Research done on tea, coffee and wine indicates that these beverages can have significant positive effects on our health.

Tea

There are hundreds of varieties of tea, but most of them fall into one of three main categories – black, green and oolong. Tea is categorized by the method used for processing the leaves. Green tea requires the least processing and black tea the most. With green tea, the leaves are immediately steamed or pan-fried and dried after picking. Black tea is fully fermented before it is pan-fried and dried, giving it a darker color, different aroma and higher caffeine content. Oolong tea is partially fermented making it stronger than green tea, but milder than black tea. Oolong tea is among the most expensive teas in the world.

Over a decade ago, Dutch scientists first found that subjects who drank tea on a regular basis had a lower incidence of heart disease and stroke. They concluded that flavonoids in green, black or oolong tea have a protective effect on the heart.

The study was done by the Netherlands National Institute of Public Health and the Environment over a 15 year period and followed 552 men. The study showed that men who drank tea had a reduced risk of stroke. Researchers concluded that the flavonoids in black tea helped reduce the production of LDL, the "bad" cholesterol that can lead to strokes and heart attacks. They wrote, "Men who drank more than 4.7 cups per day had a 69% reduced risk of stroke, compared to men who drank less than 2.6 cups per day."

A study done by Dr. Joseph Vita at Boston University School of Medicine following 66 men with coronary heart disease showed black tea can reverse abnormal functioning of the blood vessels, which could contribute to stroke. The participants in the study were given 30 ounces of tea or 30 ounces of water to drink, daily for four weeks. At the end of the month, blood vessel functioning improved by about 50% in the tea drinkers, but there was no change in those drinking water. This study also showed that there was an improvement in the functioning of the blood vessels within two hours of drinking a cup of black tea. The study was published in the journal *Circulation* in 2001.

Another study from Europe, which followed 4,807 Dutch men and women, showed that after six years the risk of heart attack dropped by 43% in those who drank more than three cups of black tea a day, compared with those who did not drink tea. The study was published in the *American Journal of Clinical Nutrition* in 2002.

More recently, researchers at University College London and Unilever Research Colworth found that tea may reduce stress hormone levels. The study was done on 75 healthy men with an average age of 33 years. The men were divided into two groups. One group of 37 men was given four cups of black tea per day for six weeks, and the second group of 38 men was given an identical tasting caffeinated drink with no active tea ingredients.

Both groups were asked to perform stressful tasks after which the researchers measured their blood pressure, cortisol levels and blood platelet levels. Both groups showed significant increase in blood pressure and heart rates during the tasks. However, 50 minutes after the tasks were complete, the cortisol levels in the men who drank tea had dropped by 47% compared to only 24% in the men who did not drink tea. Lead researcher, Professor Andrew Steptoe, from University College London said, "This has important health implications because slow recovery following acute stress has been associated with a greater risk of chronic illness, such as coronary heart disease." The study was published in the October 2006 issue of the journal *Psychopharmacology*.

Many studies show that both green tea and black tea can offer protection against various cancers. A study, published in the December 2005 issue of *Archives of Internal Medicine*, showed drinking tea everyday can significantly lower a woman's risk of ovarian cancer. Participants in the study were 61,067 Swedish women aged 46 to 76. Researchers found that women who drank two or more cups of tea a day had a 46% lower risk of ovarian cancer than those who did not drink tea. Women who averaged less than one cup of tea a day had an 18% lower risk of ovarian cancer than those who did not drink tea.

Green tea is the least processed tea, thus it provides the most flavonoids including catechins. The most abundant catechin in green tea is called epigallocatechin-3-gallate (EGCG). It has been shown to be a powerful antioxidant and is thought to be most responsible for the health benefits of tea.

A study published in the November 2005 issue of *Antiviral Research*, showed that drinking a cup of green tea a day can prevent or lessen the effects of flu. Researchers found that the catechin EGCG inhibited the replication of the influenza virus in cell cultures in all the subtypes of influenza virus tested.

Researchers at the University of Tokyo have shown that drinking green tea may increase bone mineral density. Their study included 655 women aged 60 years or older. They found that women who drank green tea five times a week or more had an average bone mineral density significantly higher than those drinking green tea less than five days a week. The researchers suspected that the catechin flavonoids in green tea provided the benefits via estrogenic effects known to build bone strength and/or induce apoptosis (suicide) in bone destroying cells called osteoclasts. This is similar to the ways that biphosphonate drugs prevent bone loss, but with none of the unpleasant side effects. The study was presented at the Osteoporosis Foundation World Congress on Osteoporosis in Toronto, Canada, on June 5, 2006.

A study, done at Japan's Tohoku University showed that green tea slowed the age–related decline in brain function seen as declining memory, cognitive impairment, dementia and Alzheimer's. The study was done with 1,003 subjects over 70 years of age, and compared their green tea intake with their mental sharpness. Drinking more than two cups of green tea each day reduced odds of cognitive impairment in both men and women by 64%. Those drinking four to six cups of green tea a week had a 38% lower risk of declines in brain function. The protective agent is thought to be the catechin, EGCG, a highly potent antioxidant. The Japanese cup of tea is 3.2 fluid ounces which is smaller than the North American tea cup. This study was published in the February 2006 issue of the *American Journal of Clinical Nutrition*.

Shinichi Kuriyama, M.D., Ph.D., of the Tohoku University School of Public Policy in Sendai, Japan, examined the relationship between green tea drinkers and death from all causes. The study began in 1994 and followed 40,530 adults ranging from age 40 to 79. Researchers found that women who drank five or more cups of green tea a day had 23% lower risk of dying from all causes, 31% lower risk of dying from cardiovascular disease and 62% lower risk of dying from stroke. In men that drank five or more cups of green tea a day, they had a 12% lower risk of dying from all causes, 22% lower risk of dying from cardiovascular disease and 42% lower risk of dying from stroke. The study was published in the September 2006 issue of the *Journal of American Medical Association*.

Wine

In the early 1990's, scientists were studying the "French Paradox", the surprising low incidence of cardiovascular disease found in France, where people consumed a high fat diet. Researchers found a 40% lower mortality rate for ischemic heart disease among people in France despite the high amount of saturated fats in their diet. Ever since this time, scientists have been studying red wine trying to pinpoint the reason.

Several studies showed that drinking two or three ounces of straight alcohol a day had a positive effect, but any more than that, and alcohol begins to have a negative effect. Studies comparing spirits, beer and wine show some effect with spirits and beer but a significant benefit to drinking red wine. Scientists began to suspect that the polyphenols in red wine, especially resveratrol, had particularly positive effects. Resveratrol is a natural substance that is found in grape skins, peanuts, some berries, such as blueberries, and in red wine. Black grapes are nature's best source of resveratrol.

Drinking one or two glasses of red wine each day may reduce inflammation, which has been linked to plaque buildup in the arteries. Researchers at Jefferson Medical College of Thomas Jefferson University in Philadelphia did a study that followed 40 healthy men who consumed two glasses (about 10 ounces) of red wine (Merlot) or 3.3 ounces of gin with dinner every day for 28 days. All the participants followed relatively the same diet and exercise plan during the study. Researchers analyzed blood samples before and after the study and found that those who drank red wine had lower levels of C-reactive protein and two other inflammatory markers. The antioxidant effects of the polyphenols found in red wine but not in gin are likely responsible for the added heart health benefits.

In the September 2000 issue of the *Annals of Internal Medicine*, Swedish researchers at the Karolinska Institute reported that light drinkers who consumed wine cut their risk of dying prematurely by almost one-third. Wine drinkers had a significantly lower risk of dying from cardiovascular disease and cancer, compared to people who did not drink at all.

Several studies show that red wine might suppress the growth of cancer cells. A study conducted by scientists at the University of Crete in Greece, showed that the phenolic compounds in red wine may slow the growth of breast cancer cells. Phenols were also shown to suppress the growth of prostate cancer cells. The results were published in the June 2000 issue of the *Journal of Cellular Biochemistry*. French scientists have found that resveratrol can slow the growth of liver cancer cells. The report was published in the July–August 2000 issue of *Oncology Reports*.

Drinking wine, particularly white wine, may benefit the lungs. A study done by the University of Buffalo on 1,555 men and women and presented to the American Thoracic Society in Atlanta on May 20, 2002, showed that drinking wine improved lung function. Holger Schunemann, M.D., Ph.D., assistant professor of medicine and social preventative medicine at the UB School of Medicine and Biomedical Sciences, commented, "Red wine in moderation has been shown to be beneficial for the heart, but in this case the relationship was stronger for white wine." Red wine also had a positive effect on breathing capability but the effect was weaker.

A more recent study, done by the researchers at Harvard Medical School and the National Institute on Aging, reports that resveratrol offsets the bad effects of a high calorie diet in mice and significantly extends their lifespan. This report was published electronically on November 1, 2006 in *Nature*. The mice in the study were fed very high doses of resveratrol, far more than a person could get by drinking red wine. Scientists warn that people should not be taking large doses of resveratrol supplements until more research is done with humans. Substances that are safe in small doses can prove to be harmful if taken in larger doses.

CHAPTER 15

Less Wholesome Food Choices

I will discuss some of the recent findings on less wholesome food choices. These should not be included in your eating plan, or at least kept to a minimum.

Trans Fats

Some fat is an essential ingredient in a healthy diet, but it must be a "good" unsaturated fat such as that found in olive oil, canola oil, nuts and avocadoes. Saturated fat, the kind that is found in red meat, cakes and some fried foods is considered a "bad" fat choice as it raises your overall cholesterol levels, which can lead to clogged arteries and heart attacks.

In saturated fats, the fat molecules have been saturated with hydrogen atoms, and in unsaturated fat some of the hydrogen atoms are missing.

The third and most harmful fat is a man–made fat called trans fat. These fats are a component of the partially hydro-genated oils used in some margarines, baked goods and restaurant foods such as french fries. In the 1970's, when studies showed that saturated fat was harmful, manufac-turers of margarines and baked goods switched to using unsaturated fats, like vegetable oil.

To make these more stable, more solid and easier to cook with, they added hydrogen to the molecules. These hydrogenated oils are packed with trans fats, which not only increases bad cholesterol but also lowers levels of the heart-protecting good cholesterol.

Trans fats have also been linked with inflammation of the arteries, which can increase the risk of stroke and heart disease.

A study done with monkeys showed that when one group of animals was fed a diet high in trans fats and another group was fed an equal amount of monounsaturated fat over a five year period, the animals that were fed the diet with the trans fats gained 5.4% more weight.

Even worse was the fact that the fat they gained was on the abdomen. Abdominal fat is linked to insulin resistance and type 2 diabetes. Trans fats may be partially to blame for the higher incidence of obesity and type 2 diabetes in younger people.

"The replacement was worse than the original," says Meir J. Stampfer, M.C., Ph.D., professor of epidemiology and nutrition at the Harvard School of Public Health. "Studies have shown that people who eat more trans fat have a higher risk for heart disease and diabetes."

It is important to read the label on the food products you are buying and to check for partially hydrogenated oil, shortening, or vegetable shortening. They are all synonyms for trans fats. These fats can be found in energy bars, hot cocoa, snack puddings, baked goods, peanut butter, tortillas, pancake mix, muffins and microwave popcorn to name just a few products.

Mandatory nutrition labeling and consumer pressure has caused many food manufacturers to reduce or eliminate trans fats. Many food products now carry the notation "no trans fats" on their packages. Almost all breads are now trans fat free. Denmark is the only country in the world to legislate trans fats, and limits them to 2% of the total fats in all foods.

New York City recently banned trans fats from restaurants. In December 2006, the officials at the Board of Health voted unanimously to order restaurants to eliminate trans fats from cooking oils by July 2007 and from all of their foods by July 2008.

It is important to read the labels of the food packages to determine if trans fats have been used.

Salt

Most North Americans consume far too much sodium. One level teaspoon of salt or 2,300 milligrams of sodium is the recommended daily allowance. According to the Center for Science in the Public Interest, the United States per capita consumption of salt increased from 2,800 milligrams in 1976 to 3,400 milligrams in 2000.

Salt is sodium chloride, and it's the sodium that can cause problems. Sodium increases blood pressure, which can increase the risk of heart attacks, strokes and kidney failure. High salt diets have been implicated in an increased risk of osteoporosis and stomach cancer.

In a recent study, researchers at Indiana University found that eating a high sodium diet can elevate your risk of exercise-induced asthma. Twenty-four people with this con-dition were divided into two groups. One group consumed a low sodium diet containing about 1,500 milligrams of sodium per day. The second group ate a diet, which contained about 9,000 milligrams of sodium a day. After exercising, those who ate the reduced salt diet experienced a 20% improvement in lung function compared to those who ate the high sodium diet. Lead researcher, Timothy Mickleborough, Ph.D., blames the salt for inducing inflammation of the airways, which reduces the flow of oxygen into the bloodstream.

Controlling your salt intake can be very hard to do. Most processed foods are loaded with salt. About 80% of the salt we eat is the salt that is added by manufacturers to prepared foods. Michael Jacobson, executive director of the Center for Science in the Public Interest, a Washington D.C. consumer health group, had research done on the sodium content of some popular foods. They found that processed cheese slices had the salt concentration of Atlantic seawater. Salt is inexpensive and makes food more palatable. It is, therefore, most often added as a flavor enhancer in processed foods.

Australian researchers found that when excessive salt is consistently added to food, our salt taste buds shrivel and become ineffective. We can no longer taste the salt and tend to over salt the food we eat. If we were to stop using salt and flavor our food with pepper, cumin, curry, garlic, spices, lemon juice, etc., our salt taste buds would grow back, and we would be able to taste the salt that's already in the food. We wouldn't be tempted to add extra.

In response to consumer demands, many manufacturers are making salt reduced products. Soups, snack foods and crackers are now available with reduced salt content. Foods that are low in sodium contain less than 140 milligrams of sodium per serving.

One gram of salt contains 400 milligrams of sodium. Our daily salt intake should be just over 5 grams or 2,300 milligrams of sodium.

Some soups can contain 1,320 milligrams of sodium in one serving, while frozen dinners can contain 4,000 to 5,000 milligrams of sodium. This is an excessive amount of sodium, considering that our daily intake should be 2,300 milligrams. You would be getting about twice your daily sodium requirement in one meal. Read the labels on the foods you buy and avoid products with excessive sodium content.

Sugar

Refined sugars are fast-digesting carbohydrates which cause blood glucose and insulin levels to spike quickly. For this reason, it is best to keep the amount of sugar consumed to a minimum.

Many foods products contain sugar. Read the labels on the foods you are buying to determine which sugars are present and in what quantity. Glucose, sucrose, fructose, lactose, maltose, corn syrup, and molasses are all sugars. Glucose is often called dextrose and it is the sugar that is most rapidly absorbed into the blood stream. Sucrose is table sugar, fructose is the main sugar found in fruits and lactose is the primary sugar found in dairy products.

Corn syrup is a sugar extracted from corn. One tablespoon of corn syrup contains twice the calories of one tablespoon of granulated sugar. Molasses is a thick syrup which is a by-product of the sugar refining process. Molasses contains some nutrients other than carbohydrates, and the darker the molasses the more nutrients. Blackstrap molasses, for instance, contains calcium, iron, potassium and traces of the B vitamins.

Brown sugar is table sugar made brown by adding molasses. Raw sugar is sometimes considered a more "natural" sugar and therefore better for you. It is, however, crystallized refined white sugar with a touch of molasses left in it. The crystals may be larger than ordinary white sugar, but it is not more natural or nutritious.

The average can of soda contains about ten teaspoons of sugar. Sugar mixed with water causes an even faster insulin spike. The liver responds by turning the excess sugar into fat.

Read the labels on foods to determine if the product contains high amounts of sugar. Cereals, soups, canned tomato paste, ketchup and bread are among the many products that contain sugar. Avoid buying foods with more than four grams of sugar per serving.

CHAPTER 16

Creating Healthy Meals and Snacks

As I mentioned earlier, it is important to balance your meals and snacks with a slow-digesting carbohydrate, a low fat protein and a small amount of desirable fat. Now that I have discussed some of the wholesome and not so wholesome food choices, we can begin to create healthy meals and snacks.

For each meal, including breakfast, have a high quality low fat protein. The portion should be about the size of your palm, this will fill one third of your plate. The other two thirds of your plate should be filled with slow-digesting carbohydrates.

I will give you a few examples of healthy meals, but you can make your own choices from the foods that you enjoy eating most.

Breakfast

- Two eggs or four egg whites scrambled with a one ounce piece of shredded low fat cheese and one cup of chopped mushrooms and onions. Add two strips of turkey bacon and a half of a honeydew melon on the side.
- One cup of slow-cooking oatmeal sprinkled with cinnamon, two tablespoons of crushed walnuts or slivered almonds and a half a cup of blueberries. Add a half of a cup of low fat cottage cheese on the side.
- A two egg omelet made with a cup of vegetables, such as asparagus, mushrooms, onions, broccoli, tomato and an ounce of finely cubed extra lean cooked ham. Choose vegetables you enjoy eating. Add half a grapefruit on the side.
- A two egg omelet with two ounces of smoked salmon, some fresh dill and one half of a cup of diced tomatoes. Add a kiwi fruit on the side.

- Two poached eggs. Add a slice of whole grain toast with a tablespoon of low fat cream cheese and an ounce of extra lean Canadian bacon. Have one half of a cup of raspberries on the side.

- French toast using one slice of whole grain bread, one egg and one ounce of shredded low fat cheese. Sprinkle with cinnamon and have one half of a cup of unsweetened applesauce on the side.

- A cup of plain low fat yogurt with one half of a cup of low fat cottage cheese and one half of a cup of sliced strawberries. Add two tablespoons of slivered almonds or crushed walnuts.

- A small whole grain bagel with three tablespoons of light cream cheese and three ounces of lox or smoked salmon.

Lunch

- A large salad using two cups of romaine lettuce or baby spinach and one cup of vegetables, such as celery, bell peppers, radishes, tomatoes, cooked green beans, etc. Add to this, a palm size piece (about four ounces) of low fat protein such as turkey, grilled chicken, lean beef, shrimp or tofu. As a dressing, use one tablespoon of vinegar and olive oil dressing. Have a pear for dessert.

■ A bean salad using one cup of romaine lettuce with one cup of cooked beans, one cup of chopped red peppers, onions and tomatoes and an ounce of low fat chicken. Use one tablespoon of vinegar and olive oil as dressing. Add an apple for dessert.

■ An open faced tuna salad sandwich using whole grain bread. Use four ounces of tuna packed in water, add chopped celery and onion to taste, add one tablespoon of relish and one quarter of a chopped green apple. Mix with one tablespoon of low fat mayonnaise. Top the sandwich with romaine lettuce and sliced tomatoes. Have a tangerine for dessert.

■ A whole grain mini pita pocket stuffed with shredded romaine, red peppers, tomatoes, onions and an ounce of shredded low fat cheese. Add three ounces of turkey breast. Have a half of a cup of cherries for dessert.

■ A palm–sized piece of poached or broiled wild salmon with a cup of coleslaw. Add a cup of blackberries for dessert.

■ Grilled turkey burger with a salad containing two cups of romaine lettuce mixed with one cup of tomatoes, onions, cucumbers and radishes. Use one tablespoon of vinegar and olive oil as dressing. Have a peach for dessert.

- Bean soup and a spinach salad with two cups of spinach, one sliced hard boiled egg and two ounces of shredded low fat cheese. One tablespoon of olive oil and vinegar as a dressing. Add a half of a cup of grapes for dessert.

- Open faced sandwich using one slice of rye bread, two ounces of lean cooked ham or lean Canadian bacon and a one ounce slice of low fat cheese. Add lettuce, tomato and onion on top. Have an apple for dessert.

Dinner

- Chicken breast (about four ounces) baked in tomato sauce with one cup of steamed broccoli served with a spinach salad containing two cups of spinach, a sliced tomato and a few slices of red onion. Use one table-spoon of olive oil and vinegar as the dressing. Have one half of a cup of strawberries and a tablet of 85% dark chocolate for dessert.

- Baked, poached or broiled wild salmon (six ounces) with 15 asparagus spears and a broiled tomato sprinkled

with low fat cheese. Serve with one half of a cup of
wild rice. Have a cup of raspberries for dessert.

- Stir-fry three cups of several different vegetables, such
  as broccoli, sweet peppers, mushrooms, green beans,
  onions, garlic or any vegetables you especially enjoy in
  one tablespoon of olive oil. Add a palm sized portion
  (about four ounces) of a low fat protein such as chicken
  or tofu. Add a pear for dessert.

- Stir-fry five ounces of shrimp with onions, garlic and
  chopped red pepper in one tablespoon of olive oil.
  Serve with one cup of zucchini and one cup of yellow
  squash. Have a cup of strawberries for dessert.

- Make a curried chicken dish with fresh ginger, garlic,
  chopped onion, fresh tomatoes, fresh cilantro or
  parsley, curry powder and pepper to taste. Add a
  palm-sized portion of stir fried cubed chicken breast.
  Serve with a cup of steamed green beans and a half of
  a cup of wild rice. Have a half of a cup of pineapple
  for dessert.

- Baked pork tenderloin (four ounce portion) with one
  cup of green beans and one cup of turnip. Add one cup
  of spinach salad with onions and tomatoes and one
  tablespoon of olive oil and vinegar dressing. Add an
  apple for dessert.

- A chicken or beef fajita using a whole grain tortilla. Fill with two cups of chopped onion, green and red peppers, tomato, four tablespoons of low fat shredded cheese and two tablespoons of guacamole. Have a tangerine for dessert.
- Baked, poached or broiled fish (six ounces) with one cup of snow peas and one half of a cup of whole grain pasta. Add a kiwi for dessert.

Healthy Snacks

Having healthy snacks, curbs your appetite, keeps your hormones balanced and provides energy. You can use any of the good carbohydrates, protein, fat combinations to create a delicious and nutritious snack. Take care not to overindulge. Eating small portions throughout the day is the best way to maintain insulin levels.

I will give you a few examples of healthy snacks, but you can be creative with the foods you like and make snacks that you enjoy and look forward to eating.

- An ounce of low fat cheese with a couple of whole grain crackers.

- An ounce of low fat cheese with a glass of wine.
- A half of a cup of low fat cottage cheese mixed with a finely chopped celery stick and green onion. Add two chopped olives.
- An ounce and a half of left over chicken, turkey or fish with a couple of olives and a small apple.
- Four tablespoons of dip made from blended chickpeas or beans. Blend beans or chickpeas with garlic, parsley, tahini and olive oil to make a nutritious dip. Have the dip with celery, red or green pepper strips, broccoli or whole wheat crackers.
- Three cooked asparagus wrapped in a slice of turkey or ham with a couple of olives.
- Remove the yolk from a hard boiled egg and stuff the egg with three tablespoons of hummus.
- One half of a cup of chopped cherry tomatoes, one ounce of crumbled low fat feta cheese and one quarter of an avocado.
- One half of a cup of cottage cheese mixed with a small finely chopped apple. Sprinkle with cinnamon and two tablespoons of slivered almonds.
- One and a half cups of plain low fat yogurt with one and a half cups of strawberries. Sprinkle with two tablespoons of crumbled walnut pieces.
- An ounce of low fat cheese with a pear.

CHAPTER 17

Organic Foods

In the past few years, organic foods have gained in popularity. The Food Marketing Institute in Washington, D.C. reported that nearly two-thirds of shoppers think organic food is healthier.

Organic foods are grown without pesticides, herbicides, hormones and antibiotics. These chemicals can eventually be absorbed by the body when the foods are consumed. The UN Food and Agricultural Organization reported in 2000 that "It has been demonstrated that organically produced foods have lower levels of pesticide and veterinary drug residues and, in most cases, lower nitrate contents."

In the European Union and the United States, organic farming is defined by law. The use of the term "organic" to describe foods and farming is regulated by the government. Presently in Canada, voluntary certification is available.

Enhancing soil health is the cornerstone of organic farming. Organic agriculture requires that the soil and the ecosystem that is used to raise the crops and livestock are kept alive with microbiotic organisms. Herbicides, pesticides and inorganic fertilizers disrupt or destroy the microbiotic activity in the soil and cannot be used in organic farming. On organic farms, livestock and poultry are grazed outdoors and are not fed hormones or antibiotics.

Skeptics of organic food say that produce on organic farms can be exposed to E. coli bacteria because organic farms mostly use manure as fertilizer. On occasion, organic foods have been implicated with contamination by E. coli bacteria. However, at times, foods that are not organically grown have also been found to be E. coli contaminated. Most manure used as a fertilizer in organic farming is composted. The high temperatures reached when manure is left in compost heaps should kill the bacteria. The manure used on organic farms is strictly regulated, and cannot be put down up to 120 days before the food is harvested.

Food safety concerns and environmental issues have made the public more aware of organic foods and organic farming. Organic foods are now becoming more in demand, and are becoming available in large grocery chain stores. For many years, organic foods could only be bought in health food stores and specialty shops at elevated prices.

The cost of organic food depends on the product. Sometimes, the difference in price is just a few pennies more. Since organic foods usually don't have as long a shelf life, it is possible to find a good buy on produce that the supermarket has bought in volume.

Foods grown organically usually cost more. Most organic farms are small and are still family–run operations. When delicate crops are grown, they are usually hand picked. Fruits are allowed to ripen on the tree, and then gently picked by hand, which will increase the cost of buying this fruit.

Non–organic apples, peaches, berries and spinach are highest in pesticides, so these may be a wise choice to buy as organic. If you can afford it, it may be better to go organic on all produce.

Most organic fruits and vegetables are about 10 to 30% higher in cost, but consumers wishing to buy chemical free organic foods are willing to spend this extra amount.

If you have a garden, you may want to try to grow some of your own organic produce. You can order organic seeds, and begin to grow them in containers or directly in your garden.

CHAPTER 18

Food or Supplements?

It is always better to get your nutrition from food rather than from supplements. Supplements do not have the life force energy that foods have, and cannot supply the large array of goodness that a living organism can. There are immeasurable benefits to eating fruits and vegetables to obtain nutrition rather than relying on supplements.

Even with today's superior technology, scientists are not able to measure all the components of food that provide health benefits. Foods contain a balance of vitamins, minerals, phytochemicals, antioxidants, fiber, etc. It is this entire combination that gives us the health benefits. Supplements cannot provide this plethora of goodness.

Foods have a complex chemistry, and contain a number of components that work individually, or together as a combination, to provide health benefits. As an example, garlic contains allium, diallyl sulfide, allyl–thiosulfinate and selenium. Studies show that garlic may protect against cancer, reduce blood pressure and reduce inflammation.

Any one of the compounds garlic contains or a combination of all of the compounds could be providing the health benefits. A garlic supplement cannot reproduce what is found in nature. Tests done on garlic supplements have shown that there is a wide variation in the compounds that are present in the supplement as well as in the concentration of these compounds. Some garlic supplements may not have enough of the correct component to provide the health benefit, while others may not have the right combination. Avoiding nutritious foods and hoping to get the same benefit from a supplement is not a wise decision.

But there are a few nutrients that we may have difficulty obtaining from food alone. Since every person's blood chemistry is different, some people may require a specific supplement, while others may not. Therefore, before taking supplements, it is best to consult with your physician.

Vitamin B6, B12 and folic acid

For many years now, scientists have been investigating B vitamins and the role they play in providing protection against heart disease, stroke and certain cancers.

Studies have shown that folic acid, a B vitamin, could provide a decreased risk of infants being born with certain birth defects, if the mothers had sufficient folic acid in their diet during pregnancy

Because of the strong evidence pointing to the protective effect of folic acid, the U.S and Canada began to fortify breads and cereals with folic acid in the late 1990's. These products are usually labeled as "enriched". Folate is the natural form of B vitamin that is found in foods, like citrus fruits and juices, whole grain products, dark leafy greens and legumes. Folic acid is the synthetic form that is found in supplements or in fortified foods.

Folic acid first came on the scene when studies showed that women, who consumed an adequate intake of folic acid before they got pregnant, decreased the risk of giving birth to a child with neural tube defects. Neural tube defects originate in the first month of pregnancy, which is before most women know that they are pregnant. It is recommended that women of child bearing age take a folic acid supplement, as many pregnancies are not planned. Severe brain and spinal birth defects have dropped by 27% in the U.S. since 1998 when folic acid was added to many foods.

Further studies on folic acid showed that it can provide other protective benefits. Researchers at the Harvard School of Public Health did a study evaluating blood plasma levels of folate, vitamins B6 and B12 with the risk of breast cancer. The study involved 32,826 nurses. The study showed that women with the highest folate levels (greater than 14ng/mL) had a 27% lower risk of breast cancer than did women with lower folate levels (less than 6.4ng/mL).

The protective effect of folic acid was even more pronounced with women who drank one or more alcoholic drinks per day. In this group, those with the highest folate levels had an 89% lower risk of breast cancer than the women with lower levels of folate. These results indicate that women who consumed a high folic acid diet reduced the risk of breast cancer that is associated with drinking alcohol. It may be a benefit for women who drink one or more alcoholic drinks per day to supplement with folic acid. The results were published in the *Journal of the National Cancer Institute* on March 5, 2003.

Folic acid, along with vitamin B6 and B12, has been shown to lower blood levels of homocysteine, an amino acid which has been associated with artery damage. Elevated homocysteine levels have been implicated in the risk of developing heart attack, stroke, peripheral vascular disease and osteoporosis.

People with high levels of homocysteine are more at risk for osteoporosis. High levels of homocysteine double the risk of osteoporosis related fractures. A report from Holland found that the risk of such fractures was twice as high in people with homocysteine levels in the top 25%, as compared to those with lower levels of homocysteine.

A report from Erasmus Medical Centre in Holland analyzed data from two studies involving a total of 2,406 people aged 55 or older. Those with the highest levels of homocysteine were 1.9 times more likely than the others to suffer osteoporosis related fractures.

A U.S. study involving 825 men and 1,174 women aged 59 to 91 found that men were four times more likely and women two times more likely to have osteoporosis related fractures when their homocysteine levels were in the top 25% as compared to those in the bottom 25%. The participants were part of the Framingham Heart Study and were followed for 12 to 15 years.

Consult with a physician before you supplement with folic acid. Excess folic acid can mask a deficiency of vitamin B12. Many people who are over 50 years of age do not absorb vitamin B12 efficiently and are deficient in this vitamin. Taking folic acid can correct anemia that is caused by folic acid deficiency, but it will not correct the underlying B12 deficiency. Permanent nerve damage can occur if the B12 deficiency is not treated.

Vitamin B12 is found in foods of animal origin such as eggs, meat, poultry, milk and fish, so many vegetarians may be at risk of a deficiency. If you are over 50 years old or a vegetarian your physician may advise you to take vitamin B12 along with the folic acid to ensure you are not deficient in this important vitamin.

There are also risks associated with taking an excess of vitamin B6. This vitamin is found in foods such as whole grains, legumes and fish. At one time, it was recommended to women with premenstrual syndrome. Women would, initially, take the recommended small doses, but if they didn't find relief they would increase the dose without consulting their physician. Some women were taking massive doses each day and began to experience pain and numbness of the extremities. It was at this time that scientists did studies and concluded that excess B6 can cause sensory nerve damage. In some cases the damage was reversible, but unfortunately, in others it was not.

It is best to consult a physician to determine whether you would benefit from B vitamins and at what dose you should be taking them.

Vitamin D

Vitamin D is produced by our body when our skin is exposed to the rays of the sun. The ultraviolet light interacts with oil in our skin producing vitamin D which is then absorbed into our body. The sun provides us with a safe and optimal supply of vitamin D. However, we have been cautioned by dermatologists about the dangers of exposing our skin to the sun. Sun exposure can cause an increased risk of skin cancer as well as having significant aging effects on our skin. Most people wear sun screen as part of their daily routine and very rarely expose their skin to the sun. Sunscreen is now found in moisturizers, make-up and body lotions to ensure that we have minimal sun exposure. However, without sun exposure we cannot produce the quantity of vitamin D we require.

Even without sunscreen, the sun must be high in the sky before we get enough ultraviolet light to produce vitamin D. By October in northern latitudes the sun is often too low in the sky to make the required amount of vitamin D. Exposing just your face and hands to ultraviolet light for a few minutes a day in northern latitudes is not sufficient.

The American Academy of Dermatology published results of a study showing that the amount of vitamin D produced when you expose your skin to sun is proportional to the amount of skin exposed. For Caucasians, most of the benefit happens within 10 minutes. Spending more time in the sun breaks down as much vitamin D as is made. There is no additional benefit to staying in the sun longer. If you lie in the sun in a bathing suit for five minutes on the front and five minutes on the back, you would produce an equivalent of 10,000 IU of vitamin D. People with darker skin color would need more time in the sun to generate the same amount of vitamin D.

Research shows that vitamin D may also play a role in preventing certain cancers. According to data from several U.S. health surveys published from the Harvard School of Public Health in 2005, vitamin D has been shown to have beneficial effects in preventing breast, prostate and other kinds of cancer. Americans who consume the highest amounts of vitamin D have a 30% lower risk of dying from cancer compared to those who consume the least amount of vitamin D.

The National Cancer Institute has mortality maps that show death rates from various cancers across the United States. Mortality from skin cancer and melanoma goes up in the Southern States with a total average mortality rate of about four people per 100,000 population. As you head north, there is a striking increase in the death rates from prostate, breast and colorectal cancers. For these cancers, the mortality rate totals about 70 per 100,000 population. This is significantly higher than rates for skin cancer and melanoma.

Bill Grant, a former NASA scientist, has combined data from cancer mortality rates with satellite measurements of ultraviolet light hitting different regions of the United States. He published graphs that show that as you move from less sunny areas such as Canada toward the ultraviolet rich areas of the southern states the decline in breast, prostate and colon cancer deaths is about 30%.

The *American Journal of Public Health* published work done by the University of California that investigated more than 60 studies that looked at the relationship between the amount of vitamin D and the risk of developing cancer. They evaluated breast, colon, prostate and ovarian cancers and found that vitamin D was protective against cancer.

Research is being done with vitamin D and autoimmune diseases, such as multiple sclerosis, type 1 diabetes and lupus. Results show that people who were born and who have lived in southern latitudes for the first ten years of their lives had decreased risk of developing multiple sclerosis during their life time, as compared to those who were born and who continued to live in northern latitudes. Other studies showed that blood levels of vitamin D were lower in those people that had multiple sclerosis than in those that did not.

Researchers from the Harvard School of Public Health analyzed blood serum samples of U.S. military personnel and found that white males with the highest levels of vitamin D were 62% less likely to develop multiple sclerosis compared with those with the lowest levels of vitamin D. The research appears in the December 20, 2006 issue of the online *Journal of the American Medical Association.*

For many years now research has shown that vitamin D plays a role in aiding calcium absorption and is important in maintaining bone health. Depending on your age, you may need more or less of this vitamin to aid with calcium absorption. Some experts believe that the best way to prevent osteoporosis is to have children develop their bone mass at an early age. They feel it may be wise to supplement children with a small dose of vitamin D.

The verdict by many experts is that we don't consume enough vitamin D. Dr. Michael Holick, a researcher at Boston University, calls the vitamin D shortage "an epidemic" in North America and Europe. Experts are suggesting an increase in the recommended daily levels of vitamin D from 400 IU to 1000 IU or more. Some research has shown that to prevent fractures, older adults should take 2,000 IU of vitamin D a day.

Few foods supply vitamin D, so meeting your quota with foods alone can be difficult. You can find vitamin D in fish, such as salmon, sardines, mackerel, canned tuna, in egg yolk and fortified products such as milk, juices and some cereals. It is also difficult to get your quota through sun exposure if you live in northern climates or if you continually wear sunscreen.

Vitamin D exists in several forms that have different activity levels. Vitamin D3, cholecalciferol, is the most active form of vitamin D and is the form required for retaining bone density. It is potent in small quantities. One microgram of cholecalciferol has 40 IU of vitamin D activity.

It is best to consult with your physician to determine if you or your family requires vitamin D and the dosage that you should be taking.

Calcium

Calcium is the most common mineral found in our body. About 99% of the calcium is found in our teeth and bones while the other 1% is found in the blood and soft tissue. Our body maintains the calcium levels in our blood within a narrow range. If the calcium drops below this level, our body takes the calcium from our bones. In order to maintain healthy bones, we require a sufficient amount of calcium in our diet, otherwise, we will suffer debilitating consequences as we age.

Osteoporosis is a disease in which the bone mass diminishes to a point that bone fractures easily occur. It can affect women, men and children; however, osteoporosis is most frequently diagnosed in postmenopausal women. Sustaining a hip fracture is one of the most serious consequences of osteoporosis in older people. One out of five people die within a year of sustaining the fracture.

Increased age, female gender, smoking, estrogen deficiencies and certain medications are factors that increase the risk of osteoporosis. To reduce the risk of being diagnosed with osteoporosis it is wise to attain peak bone mass during youth and then try to maintain it with age. Exercise as well as sufficient calcium intake is critical for every age group. Young women who avoid dairy products might be wise to take calcium supplements to build up their bone mass early on.

Supplemental calcium alone can't restore bone loss in individuals with osteoporosis. However, if drug therapy is recommended, an adequate amount of calcium is needed along with vitamin D and magnesium. The usual recommended dose of calcium is 1,200 milligrams a day, along with 600 to 1,000 milligrams of vitamin D and 600 milligrams of magnesium.

If you do take calcium supplements, to maximize absorption do not take more than 600 milligrams of calcium at a time. It is best to take one tablet in the morning and one in the evening. Consult with your physician to determine if you require a calcium supplement and the amount that you require.

Magnesium

The metabolic role of magnesium is very diverse and it affects almost every body system we have. Our cardiovascular system, digestive system, nervous system, brain, kidneys, liver, glands and muscles rely on magnesium.

Minerals activate enzymes and over 300 enzyme functions depend on magnesium including the enzyme that generates energy for all our body cells. Magnesium is involved in metabolizing fats, proteins and carbohydrates. It aids in proper functioning of genes, DNA synthesis and cell replication. It is required for energy production, muscle relaxation, cardiovascular health, maintaining bone density and aiding with the absorption of other minerals such as calcium and potassium.

Maintaining adequate magnesium levels is especially important to people who have type 2 diabetes and cardiovascular disease. People with insulin resistance usually have low levels of magnesium in their tissues. Dr. Jerry Nadler, division chief of endocrinology and metabolism at the University of Virginia in Charlottesville, put 16 healthy people on magnesium deficient diets for three weeks. The results showed that not only did their cells become deficient in magnesium, but their insulin was less capable of transporting the blood glucose into their cells. He remarked, "You can induce insulin resistance even in people who do not have diabetes. Just deprive them of magnesium."

Dr. Nadler found that people with type 2 diabetes not only had a deficiency in magnesium, but had twice as much of the blood clotting factor thromboxane as people without the disease. Supplementing with magnesium may help reduce the thromboxane levels, and thereby, reduce the amount of vascular disease in patients with diabetes.

Magnesium may play a role in managing high blood pressure. Lawrence Resnick, M.D., professor of medicine and director of hypertension at Wayne State University School of Medicine in Detroit, measured magnesium levels in people with type 2 diabetes and without diabetes. He found that people with diabetes had significantly lower magnesium levels and higher blood pressure than those without the disease. He also found that people with high blood pressure, whether they were diabetic or not, had lower levels of magnesium. "I have treated people who were hypertensive and on one or two medications with magnesium," says Dr. Resnick. "Their blood pressure is normal now."

Some experts believe insufficient magnesium may play a role in heart disease, hypertension, diabetes, asthma, abdominal obesity, migraines, muscle pains, infertility, pre-menstrual syndrome and stress.

"Not getting the right amount of magnesium is a growing concern for everyone – it's vital to overall health, especially for those people with certain medical conditions," says "Dr. Andrea Rosanoff, who has spent 17 years studying magnesium. She is co-author of the book *The Magnesium Factor* along with Dr. Mildred Seelig, who spent 35 years studying the role of magnesium in health.

Large amounts of magnesium can be lost during prolonged exercise, excessive sweating or when using diuretics. Magnesium deficiency can cause muscle twitching, leg cramps, depression, nausea, migraines, dizziness, abnormal heart rhythms, spasms of the coronary arteries, blood clots and high blood pressure.

If you are eating the typical North American diet that includes large amounts of highly processed foods, then you may not be getting enough magnesium. Magnesium is available in foods such as whole grain breads and cereals, brown rice, cashews, almonds, bananas, orange juice, black beans, kidney beans, pinto beans, spinach, broccoli and fish such as pollock, tuna, flounder and sardines.

A proper balance must be maintained between calcium and magnesium to ensure proper use of both these minerals. If you take calcium supplements without magnesium, you may be distorting this balance. The ratio of calcium to magnesium should be two to one. If you consume 1,000 milligrams of calcium per day then you would need 500 milligrams of magnesium.

Renal failure patients should not take magnesium supplements. As with any supplement, consult with your doctor to determine if you should be taking magnesium and at what dose.

Omega-3 Fatty Acids

Omega-3 fats are a group of unsaturated essential fatty acids. Researchers began to focus on the benefits of omega-3 in the early 1980's when studies showed that Greenland Eskimos whose diets were rich in omega-3 fatty acids had very low rates of heart disease. Since then, scientists have linked these fats to assorted health benefits.

An important finding was that omega-3 fats reduce inflammation. Inflammation has been implicated in increasing the risk of type 2 diabetes, Alzheimer's, irritable bowel syndrome, macular degeneration, rheumatoid arthritis, asthma, autoimmune disorders, heart disease and several cancers.

Omega–3 fats provide a variety of benefits for the heart. They reduce the levels of triglycerides, LDL cholesterol and decrease the risk of blood clots that can lead to a heart attack or stroke.

Researchers from the Harvard School of Public Health found that eating a moderate amount of fish a week, about three ounces of salmon or six ounces of mackerel, reduced the risk of death from coronary heart disease, but also reduced the overall rate of death from all causes. The paper appeared in the October 18, 2006 issue of the *Journal of the American Medical Association*.

In this study, researchers also addressed the concerns of the potential harmful effects to humans from chemicals found in fish. They looked at the benefit of fish consumption as well as the health risks from mercury, PCB's and dioxins. They focused on cardiovascular health in adults and brain development in infants. The evidence across different studies showed that moderate fish consumption lowers the risk of death from heart disease by 36%. The lead author of the study, Dariush Mozaffarian, said, "Overall, for major health outcomes among adults, the benefits of eating fish greatly outweigh the risks."

Researchers found no definite evidence that low level mercury exposure from eating fish had harmful effects on the health of adults. They did find that mercury may lessen the cardiovascular benefit, but eating fish did not cause net harm.

Mozaffarian commented, "We also found that fish or fish oil intake reduces total mortality by 17%, a remarkable reduction considering that this is the benefit for deaths from all causes."

For infants and young children, the authors found that omega-3 fatty acids likely improve brain development. There had been some concern that mercury can have a detrimental affect on brain development. The investigator's findings agreed with the Environmental Protection Agency that young children and nursing mothers should eat up to two servings a week of a variety of fish, such as salmon, light tuna, mackerel or shrimp. Only four species of fish should be avoided – golden bass, king mackerel, shark and swordfish which are larger fish and would have higher mercury levels. This advisory is only for children and pregnant and nursing mothers, and not for the general public.

The study points out that only 9% of the PCB's and dioxins in the food supply come from fish and more than 90% comes from dairy products, vegetables and meats.

Because of the recent press on the many benefits of omega-3 fats, products such as milk, yogurt, eggs and juices, have started to appear on the shelf with omega-3 added.

Caution must be taken with some of these products. For instance, in the case of omega-3 eggs, the hens diet could include plant sources rich in omega-3 such as flaxseed, but the hens could also be fed a diet of fish meal yielding the same kind of omega-3 as found in fish. Although these eggs may be nutritious, there may be some concern with feeding hens fish meal. Some scientists question the wisdom of using a feed made from another species to produce food rich in omega-3. Other problems could arise, such as Creutzfeldt-Jacob disease, also known as mad cow disease.

Our body is unable to make omega-3 so we must obtain it from food or a supplement. Omega-3 fats are found in cold water fish, such as salmon, herring, sardines and mackerel. Alpha-linolenic acid (ALA) is the omega-3 found in plant foods, such as flaxseeds, walnuts, canola, avocado and leafy greens. If you are not eating foods rich in omega-3, then you may want to consider taking an omega-3 supplement. Because of the numerous health benefits many scientists believe that everyone should supplement with omega-3 regardless of their diet.

If you decide to take a supplement of omega-3, consult with your physician for the dosage you should be taking. Also if you are taking fish oil, it is best to buy a pharmaceutical grade that does not contain contaminants such as

PCB's, dioxins or heavy metals. Be aware that supplements such as cod liver oil may contain an excess of vitamin A and much less omega-3 than salmon oil.

CHAPTER 19

What Can Sabotage the Perfect Eating Plan?

Falling off the Wagon

It is important not to get discouraged if you "fall off" your eating plan from time to time. Many people think all is lost when they slip off a diet. They become discouraged and may go back to their less healthy eating habits.

The perfect eating plan is not a restrictive diet. It is a healthy way of eating. It is a way of balancing meals to keep your glucose and insulin levels in check. This will keep your weight in control and your health at its peak.

Try to balance your food intake with a protein, slow-digesting carbohydrate and good fat. You will not have a disastrous result if you don't do this from time to time. Keep your meals balanced as much as possible, and if you slip occasionally, just go back to balancing your next meal or snack.

Cravings

Harvey Weingarten, Ph.D., president and vice-chancellor of the University of Calgary in Alberta conducted extensive research on food cravings and found that 97% of women and 68% of men have felt cravings. He commented, "Cravings are a natural part of our relationship to food." We give in to our cravings at least half the time.

It is better to satisfy a craving in moderation than to deny it and later overeat to compensate. If we deny our cravings every time, we might begin to feel deprived. We might be more likely to abandon healthy eating habits. It is important to have a treat that you crave from time to time. If you are craving a sweet, then having some protein with the sweet will slow down the production of insulin.

If you are craving a dessert, rate the dessert for tastiness. Is it worth the calories? Do you love it that much? If you're not crazy about the dessert, then don't eat it, as it is not worth the calories or the havoc that it will play with your insulin levels. If you crave some decadent chocolate cake and love the taste and feel it is worth the calories, then enjoy a small piece without guilt.

Cravings are specific and people usually crave a certain food, such as donuts, chips or sweets. Keep these foods out of your home so you won't be tempted when you're craving strikes. You can substitute a healthier snack, such as whole grain crackers with cheese, vegetables with cheese, whole grain pita with hummus or fruit with yogurt. If you are craving for a sweet or chocolate then a piece of dark 85% chocolate might satisfy your craving and also give you some health benefits.

Many times cravings hit us when we are stressed out, upset or bored. We imagine that the food we are craving will bring us comfort. Try to seek consolation another way, such as calling a friend, going for a walk or arranging to have a massage.

If your craving is persistent than denying it every time will make the urge more intense. Allow yourself a moderate portion of the food you crave but decide on the amount you will have before you begin eating.

Food Addictions

Food can be as addictive as drugs. Mr. Jaideep Bains, a neu-roscientist and assistant professor at the University of Calgary, did a presentation at The Alberta Obesity Summit, a two day seminar bringing together scientists from North America to discuss the growing obesity problem. "It's not drugs and alcohol that are the drug of choice these days – it's food", said Mr. Bains. "Feeding behaviors are not dissimilar to addictive behaviors."

Mr. Bains also noted that stress appears to be linked to eating and addiction. "Stress could make cravings (for food and drugs) more profound", he said. "There is also some thinking that it could relieve stress."

Food may have more addictive properties than people realize. Eating and drugs activate the same regions of the brain. Sweets, chocolate and salty snacks seem to be high on the addiction list. If you find you are eating large amounts of certain fast-digesting carbohydrates during the day, such as cookies or chips, then you may try to wean yourself off these slowly. Do not buy these products and bring them home where you can be tempted by them.

Beverages

Soft drinks, fruit juices and alcohol are high caloric drinks and can easily sabotage your eating plan. Consuming several glasses of these drinks daily can contribute excessive calories without satiating your hunger. Drinking water or unsweetened tea and coffee will provide benefits to your health without the calories.

Many people are simply unaware of the excessive number of calories they consume through drinks alone. A fancy cocktail has the same number of calories as a slice of pizza.

Be aware of the beverages you consume and especially the beverages that cause a spike in your glucose and insulin levels. These are the beverages that will have detrimental effects on your health and cause weight gain.

Restaurant Meals

Eating out at restaurants can sabotage your diet. Restaurants tend to serve enormous portions. A typical restaurant meal in the U.S. has at least 60% more calories than the average meal made at home according to NPD Group, a market research firm.

Research published in the *American Journal of Clinical Nutrition* in the fall of 2002, showed that portion size affects the amount of food consumed at a single meal and contributes to the increasing prevalence of obesity in the U.S.

A study conducted at the University of Pennsylvania on the effects of portion size on overall food intake found that large restaurant portions may significantly affect obesity. Both men and women in the study ate more in response to larger portions. Fewer than one half of the men and women reported they noticed a difference in the portion sizes they were given. Researchers suggest that people have the expectation that the amount of food served to them by others is appropriate. They suggest limiting portion size at restaurants and at home to slow the increasing incidence of obesity.

To keep portion size manageable at a restaurant, consider sharing the appetizer and dessert or having an appetizer as a main course. Another option is to take part of the meal home to have as a snack the following day or leave some food on the plate. Some people will continue to eat even when they are not hungry in order to finish the food on the plate.

When ordering in restaurants try to avoid fried foods and try to avoid bread. Most restaurants provide a basket of bread or rolls before the meal. If you are hungry, then you will dive into the bread basket to satisfy your hunger. White bread and rolls are fast-digesting carbohydrates that will cause a rapid increase in glucose and insulin levels.

It is best to avoid the bread and have an appetizer that has a balance of protein, carbohydrate and fat. A few shrimp with olives or a goat cheese salad would not cause insulin levels to skyrocket. If you enjoy having a piece of bread, dip it in vinegar and olive oil instead of smearing it with butter to reduce saturated fats and add the protective benefits of olive oil.

Part III

EXERCISE

CHAPTER 20

Why Exercise?

Recently, there has been much press that people, especially children, are becoming less active and are gaining far more weight than ever before. Our lives and our children's lives are becoming sedentary. Much more time is spent in front of televisions and computers and much less time is spent on physical activity.

Studies indicate that overweight children will become overweight adults. Young adults are now being diagnosed with obesity and type 2 diabetes in record numbers. In just over a decade, diabetes nearly doubled in the adult North American population, from 4.9% in 1990 to 8.7% in 2002. Obesity is becoming a costly health problem that is leading to serious illness and decreased life expectancies.

Making a lifelong commitment to a lifestyle that emphasizes proper nutrition and regular physical activity will maintain a healthy and powerful body through old age. Your chances of living an active and independent life into your sixties, seventies and eighties would improve enormously by simply staying active and eating properly. Research shows that even people in their seventies and eighties enjoy many health benefits from exercise. It's never too late to start.

It is far easier to live this improved lifestyle than it is to constantly struggle with different fad diets and exercise programs that promise instant weight loss and fitness. Most of us learn very quickly that there is no such thing as a quick fix. Many times, these regimes can do more harm than good. It is better to stay in good health and fitness rather than to try to regain your fitness level after letting it slip away.

Physical activity provides a host of benefits for everyone, but especially if you are overweight and trying to shed body fat; then regular exercise is a key to success. Exercising while losing weight helps to target body fat and protects against muscle loss. It is most important to preserve muscle, as muscle increases the metabolic rate over time, which allows us to burn more calories.

If you are highly overweight, establishing a healthy diet is the most important first step. You cannot hope to lose weight and get your hormone levels in balance with exercise alone. Once your hormone levels are in balance through proper diet, your physician can recommend an exercise program appropriate to your fitness level.

Whether you are overweight or not, proper diet is a must before you can completely enjoy the benefits of exercise. I have a friend who is an avid runner, is very lean, does core exercises and has a conditioned cardiovascular system. He also enjoyed eating many servings a day of high glycemic carbohydrates, such as white bread, pizza, pasta and candy. These cause a rapid increase in insulin and glucose levels. He felt he could consume these foods as he was "burning them off".

He had no concerns of weight gain because of his active running schedule and presumed that he was in top physical condition. He was surprised to be diagnosed with high glucose levels that, if not controlled, would lead to type 2 diabetes. He changed his diet, eliminating the high glycemic carbohydrates, and within a few months, his glucose levels dropped back to normal. A combination of proper diet and regular exercise is required to keep our hormones in balance.

Benefits of Physical Activity

It is necessary for everyone to add regular activity to their life, whether they are overweight or not. People who are active and exercise regularly reduce their risk of developing and dying from some of the leading causes of illness in North America. Physical activity can improve your mental health as well as your physical health. Being physically active:

- Reduces the risk of dying prematurely
- Reduces the risk of developing high blood pressure
- Helps lower blood pressure in people with high blood pressure
- Reduces the risk of developing high cholesterol
- Reduces the risk of developing heart disease and stroke
- Reduces the risk of developing diabetes
- Lowers excess blood glucose
- Lowers excess insulin
- Maintains healthy muscles, bones and joints
- Helps maintain proper body weight by increasing your metabolism
- Helps decrease body fat and reduces risk of obesity
- Reduces stress and helps prevent depression
- Reduces risk of developing osteoporosis
- Reduces some of the effects of aging
- Helps you sleep better
- Increases your energy and endurance

■ Reduces the risk of breast cancer. A study done in October 2003 by the University of Southern California and the American Cancer Association, and published in the journal *Cancer*, showed that women who exercised had a 35% lower risk of developing breast cancer in situ than did inactive women.

How Much Exercise Do We Need?

Although a sedentary life is not healthy, an overly aggressive exercise regime is not healthy either. A study that examined mortality rates over a 22 to 26 year period of 17,000 men, who had attended Harvard University, showed life expectancy was about two years longer for those that expended at least 2,000 calories per week compared to individuals who were sedentary.

The study, done by Stanford University's Dr. Paffenbarger, showed that the death rate declined as the number of calories burned in activity increased, but only to a point. Death rates leveled off and then began to go up again in the men that expended more than 3,000 calories per week. The optimum amount of calories that should be burned during exercise per week is 2,000 calories. That translates to about

300 calories per day. It doesn't matter what exercise you do to burn these calories.

Moderate exercise is the best way to achieve a good fitness level and longevity. The Harvard study shows that more exercise is not always better. As you increase exercise intensity, your body will be making more free radicals and cortisol which has a negative effect on longevity. Even though you are becoming more fit with longer bouts of exercise, the increased amount of free radicals and cortisol you are producing will cause you to live a shorter life.

For most people, walking briskly for a half an hour a day will provide the required amount of physical activity. Physical activity is any movement that uses energy. We don't have to belong to a gym to get exercise. We can sneak a lot of activity into our day without having a structured exercise program. We can:

- Walk to work or park the car at a distance and walk the rest of the way
- Go for a walk at lunch
- Do an activity you enjoy such as gardening
- Do housework at a fast pace
- Use the stairs instead of an elevator
- Walk to the store to do your shopping instead of driving
- Walk around a shopping mall in inclement weather

Arthritis and Exercise

It is very important to stay active as we age. Exercise gives us mobility and the ability to remain independent and cope on our own for a longer period of time.

Findings published in the journal, *Arthritis & Rheumatism*, showed that even a modest amount of exercise is better than no exercise when it comes to preventing disability from arthritis. The two year study followed more than 3,500 adults aged 53 to 63 who had osteoarthritis. The participants were divided into three groups:

- an inactive group
- insufficiently active group
- a group that got at least 30 minutes of moderate activity, such as walking or gardening on most days of the week, or 20 minutes of vigorous exercise, such as running or swimming

Overall, adults in the moderately active group were 41% less likely to show functional decline than those that were inactive. The risk reduction was almost as great for those in the insufficiently active group. Modest levels of exercise can help prevent disability from arthritis, or perhaps reverse it in some cases, according to Dr. Joe Feinglass, the study's lead author.

How to Stay Active

- Do an exercise that you find fun to do. You can get exercise by dancing, walking, cycling, in-line skating, golfing, playing tennis, gardening, swimming or any other activity that you enjoy.
- Do an exercise you are physically able to do. For people with arthritis or osteoporosis, swimming or walking may be a better exercise than a more active sport, such as tennis or squash.
- Find a friend to exercise with. People are more likely to exercise regularly and with more intensity when they have a buddy to work out with who will encourage and motivate them.
- Do an exercise routine at the gym on a regular basis.
- Take yoga classes. For a sedentary person, yoga may be a good introduction to exercise. Yoga promotes a sense of well-being and encourages commitment and discipline which will help in making lifestyle changes.
- Don't exercise if you are in pain. The "no pain, no gain" motto is a falsehood. Some muscle soreness is normal when starting an exercise program, but pain is not normal. Working through pain could cause a major injury. Stop exercising if you are in pain and consult with your doctor.

■ Don't get discouraged. It will take weeks for you to notice a change in your body once you begin to exercise regularly. If you have the desire to improve, you will.

Make Exercise a Habit

You may be more likely to exercise regularly if you set aside a certain time of day for exercise. If you are a morning person, you may wish to exercise every morning before work. If you are an afternoon person, you may feel more comfortable exercising at the same time each day after work.

Some people are more committed to exercise if they join a health club and attend aerobic, spinning, yoga or weight training classes.

It may help to keep a log of your progress. You may feel more committed to exercise if you actually see the improvements that you are making in body measurement, blood pressure, heart rate, etc.

CHAPTER 21

Condition All Systems

As mentioned before, an ideal exercise program will burn about 300 calories a day. This is not an excessive amount of activity. The most beneficial fitness program will condition our heart and lungs (aerobic exercise), strengthen our body core and maintain our muscle mass (anaerobic exercise).

If we do only aerobics, then we are only addressing one facet of our total fitness. The human body is composed of multiple systems such as cardiovascular, muscular, skeletal, nervous, circulatory, to name only a few. To be healthy and fit, you need to be aware of the need to condition all of these systems.

This may seem overwhelming if you are a beginner or don't have the time to spend on exercise, but you can do this in as little as half an hour a day, four to five days a week. You can do this at home without special equipment.

I will discuss the benefits of aerobic and core exercises, as well as strength training.

Benefit of Aerobic Exercise

Aerobic exercise improves the cardiovascular and cardiorespiratory system (heart and lungs). We breathe more deeply and the heart pumps more blood when the large muscle groups are exercised aerobically. Aerobic exercise:

- Lowers heart rate
- Lowers blood pressure
- Decreases blood triglycerides
- Increases HDL (good) cholesterol
- Reduces body fat
- Improves weight control
- Improves glucose tolerance
- Reduces chance of developing insulin resistance
- Increases blood supply to muscles

In terms of heart health, the amount of exercise that we do seems to be more important than the intensity of the exercise. A study, done at Duke University Medical Center with overweight sedentary men and women, showed that even mild exercise improved fitness and reduced cardio-vascular risk. Lead study author was Brian Duscha, an exercise physiologist at Duke University Medical Center's Division of Cardiology.

The study involved 133 people who did not exercise, were overweight, did not smoke, had rising levels of cholesterol and were 40 to 65 years of age. These people were separated into four individual exercise groups:

- High amount at high intensity – Jogging 20 miles per week
- Low amount at high intensity – Jogging 12 miles per week
- Low amount at moderate intensity – Walking briskly 12 miles per week
- Control group of people who did not exercise

Each participant had cardiopulmonary testing before the start of the study and at the end of the study after exercising for seven to nine months.

All groups that exercised saw improvements in their fitness level, but the group that did 12 miles at vigorous intensity was not significantly different to the group that did 12 miles at moderate intensity. This study shows that you get aerobic conditioning gains from brisk walking for half an hour, three or four times a week. This would be an ideal place to start for a person who is overweight or hasn't exercised for a long time.

Increasing the amount of exercise from 12 miles a week to 20 miles a week provides even more cardiovascular benefits. Duscha concludes, "It is appropriate to recommend mild exercise to improve fitness and reduce cardiovascular risk, yet encourage higher intensities and amounts for additional benefits."

Many people are reluctant to exercise thinking they will never be able to keep up with the amount of exercise that is needed to improve their health. To some people who are out of shape, the thought of having to do strenuous exercise regimes to become fit is so overwhelming that they become discouraged and don't exercise.

Duscha said, "The classic question always is: What's the minimum amount of exercise I need to do to get a health benefit." For those who are hesitant to exercise regularly, the recommendation of doing a brisk walk three or four times a week to see health benefits is a manageable goal.

Benefits of Core Body Strength

Core exercises strengthen the muscles that support the spine from the lower back to the upper back both in the front and back of the body. The core includes the pelvis, abdominal, chest and back muscles. The body core provides the basis of every movement whether it's walking or reaching for the newspaper. If the core is not properly conditioned your movements and physical abilities will be limited.

A strong base allows your body to perform at maximum potential. Even if you participate in a sport, or weight lift, you may not be conditioning the core muscles. You may be building up the biceps and triceps, but you are ignoring all the vital small muscles that support the torso, hips, shoulders and back. You will limit your physical abilities if your core is not properly conditioned. Each movement you make originates from the core. A conditioned core:

- Increases balance
- Helps improve stamina
- Helps avoid muscle strain
- Improves strength and mobility

Benefits of Strength Training

Strength training builds muscle mass that is necessary for us to preserve strength, balance and functional ability. Strength training:

- Increases muscle, tendon and ligament strength
- Reduces body fat and increases lean muscle mass
- Improves cholesterol readings
- Decreases blood pressure in some people
- Improves strength, balance and functional ability in older individuals
- Improves glucose tolerance
- Reduces chance of developing insulin resistance
- Increases bone density

STRETCHING

Over the years, many coaches and fitness experts have ingrained in their athletes and students, that stretches are an important part of exercise. The common thinking has been that stretches should be done before and after exercise to prevent injury. Recently, there has been some controversy about whether to stretch at all, and if you do stretch, whether to stretch before or after exercise.

Stephen B. Thacker M.D., director of the epidemiology program office at the Centers for Disease Control and Prevention (CDC; Atlanta, Georgia), conducted a study that reviewed 361 research studies on stretching. The conclusion was that there was no evidence that stretching before and after exercise prevents injury or muscle soreness. The results were published in the March 2004 issue of *Medicine & Science in Sports & Exercise (MSSE)*.

The study concluded that stretching does improve flexibility, but being flexible doesn't prevent injuries. Injury rates were higher for both the most flexible and the least flexible participants than they were for the participants with average flexibility. Most injuries occur when the muscle is going through the normal range of motion, so being more flexible has no effect on preventing these injuries. In fact, an increased range of motion at a joint can make it more unstable, which may account for the higher number of injuries in the most flexible participants in this study.

It is difficult to discredit this review since it included 361 studies and each of these followed hundreds or thousands of participants. The studies were also weighted so the weaker studies were given less consideration than the more rigorous ones.

The CDC review concluded that there wasn't sufficient evidence to recommend that people stretch or stop stretching to prevent injury during exercise. If you like stretching, then continue to stretch, if you don't, then put some time into warm up exercises instead.

Good conditioning is the best way to prevent injury and muscle soreness after exercise. If you continue to do the core exercises, aerobic exercises and strength training exercises that I recommend five or six times a week, then you will be in good condition and be less likely to get injured. It is necessary to be consistent. Neglecting exercise for several weeks and then starting up again at an advanced level is a sure way to cause injury.

Although stretching may not be important before exercise, a warm up is critical. A warm up increases muscle temperature, which decreases the risk of muscle and tendon injury and stiffness. Warming up consists of at least ten minutes of low level activity. Doing core exercises before aerobic activity or strength training would be a perfect way to warm up your muscles.

While this CDC study evaluated stretching with regard to injury prevention during exercise and saw no benefit, I still encourage everyone to stretch in order to relax and lengthen tense muscles. Stretching might not reduce the risk of injury during exercise, but it may reduce the risk of other injuries, such as repetitive strain injuries. Stretching elongates muscles, tendons and ligaments and keeps them flexible. As we age, tendons and ligaments become shorter, limiting our range of motion. A supervised yoga class may be a good training ground to learn correct stretching techniques.

If you do stretch, a ten minute warm up is essential. Stretching cold muscles can cause injury. Don't bounce, but hold the position until you feel a gentle pull on your muscle. Never stretch an injured muscle or hold a painful stretch. How long you hold the stretch depends on your age and physical condition. In order to prevent injury and get the most out of stretching, you should have your routine customized to your needs. It is best to consult with a fitness trainer to develop a stretching program specific to you, and give you the proper instruction on how the stretches should be done and when to do them.

How Do You Get Started?

It is important to talk with your doctor before getting started. You should know the physical condition that you are in before you begin exercising. This is especially important if you have health problems, are obese, are elderly, are pregnant or have not exercised for a long period of time.

If you have been inactive, but otherwise are in good health, start out slowly. Begin with a 15 minute period of light exercise or a brisk walk, and then gradually increase the intensity and time.

You need to make a commitment to yourself to add daily activity to your life. You receive the most benefit and the least injuries if you maintain your fitness level with regular activity.

Try not to set any preconceived limits on what you can do and try not to make excuses such as time limitations. You may feel a little challenged in the beginning, but you will eventually see the benefits.

As regular activity becomes part of your life, it will seem less of a chore and will become part of your lifestyle. Exercise will improve the quality of your life and maintain your youthfulness.

CHAPTER 22

The Perfect Exercise Plan

If you incorporate everything I have discussed thus far, you can build a perfect exercise plan specific to you. The perfect exercise plan will include an activity that:

- Consumes about 300 calories a day
- Conditions the cardiovascular system, core and maintains muscle mass
- Does not require special equipment
- Does not cause pain or injury

Anyone who is overweight or just beginning to exercise after a long period of inactivity should not be overwhelmed.

You can design your own exercise schedule that fits in with your life and fitness level.

I will make suggestions on how to condition the cardio-vascular system, the core and muscles that both beginners and intermediates can do. If you gradually work up to the intermediate level of exercise and continue to do these exer-cises on a regular basis, you will remain in good physical condition.

When your fitness level improves to the point that you are no longer challenged by these exercises, and you feel you would like a more advanced exercise program, then consult with a fitness trainer. They will provide you with proper exercises and techniques. Proper technique will prevent injury.

CARDIOVASCULAR

Cardiovascular Conditioning for Beginners

As I mentioned earlier, a study done at Duke University Medical Center found that improvements were made in aerobic conditioning in people who walked only twelve miles a week at moderate intensity. If you are just beginning to exercise or have been inactive for a long period of time, the best place to start is by walking at least three or four times a week for up to 30 minutes at moderate intensity. If you are only able to do 10 minutes at first, this is fine; you can gradually increase your time to 30 minutes.

When you feel comfortable with this amount of exercise, you can increase the amount of walking to five or six days a week at moderate intensity. This would be sufficient to keep your cardiovascular system conditioned.

This is not a daunting task. There are many ways to squeeze in your daily activity. You can walk to do errands, such as shopping or banking, instead of taking the car. Some days, you can replace your walking with another activity, such as gardening, swimming, playing golf or doing your house cleaning.

It is important to do an activity at a moderate intensity for at least half an hour. You can adjust your exercise regime to fit in with your lifestyle. Don't consider it an overwhelming chore that has to be done, but an activity that is part of your daily routine, such as brushing your teeth.

Work up to at least 30 minutes of activity at a moderate intensity for at least five or six days a week. This is not a big investment in time, and can fit into even the tightest of schedules.

Cardiovascular Conditioning for Intermediates

Some people can get addicted to exercise and invest long hours working out. This is not necessary and can actually have some negative consequences. Research, done on Harvard Alumni, showed that an overly aggressive exercise regime can cause a decrease in longevity. The study showed that exercise that burns over 400 calories a day can cause a shortened lifespan. It is believed that excessive exercise causes free radical and cortisol formation, which has a negative effect on longevity.

Burning 300 calories a day is all that is required to condition the cardiovascular system and live a long life. You can do any activity that you want to meet this requirement. Walking briskly for 30 minutes a day is a perfect exercise. If you prefer; you can play a sport such as golf and tennis, garden, swim, jog, cycle, in-line skate or go to the gym and use the treadmill, stationery bicycle or cross trainer to get your 30 minutes of activity each day.

If you continue to do 30 minutes of cardiovascular exercise, at a moderate intensity, five or six days a week, you will remain in good condition. If you wish to do a more advanced cardiovascular program, consult with a fitness instructor to get the proper exercise and techniques.

CORE EXERCISES

Each movement you make, whether it is playing a sport or whether it is doing household chores, originates from the body core. The body core is the area from the groin to the shoulders. You cannot ignore these vital muscles that support the torso, hips, shoulders and back. Your activities will be limited if your body core is not properly conditioned.

Core exercises are extremely important for every age group. They keep our bodies balanced and more powerful. You can become a better golfer, runner, tennis player or gardener, have less back injuries, have better posture and have better balance if the core area of the torso is strong.

It is amazing how quickly and painlessly this can happen. A colleague of mine enjoys jogging daily, and at times runs marathons. He has always been very thin, but he had concerns that his overall strength and flexibility were not where he would like them to be.

He began doing core exercises for 10 minutes before each run. He had anticipated that it would take months before he would see any improvements and he wasn't quite sure what these improvements would be. He was consistent in doing some core exercises every time before a run, but some days he would do less than other days.

One morning, only a few weeks later, he was getting up from the floor after doing his core exercises and he touched his abdomen. He was surprised at how hard it had become with such little effort. He mentioned that he had never been this "buff" before. The 10 minute investment that he made had paid off hugely for him. He is pleased with the results and continues to do these same core exercises before a run.

I will describe a few core exercises that will help condition this vital area of the body.

Core Exercises for Beginners

The following exercises will provide balance, core strength and stability. Begin slowly to allow your body to become accustomed to this new activity. Never hold your breath while doing these exercises. You may find them difficult to do at first, but if you persevere, you will be surprised how quickly and painlessly you will advance.

If you are unable to do ten repetitions of each exercise at the beginning, do as many as you can and gradually work up to ten repetitions. These exercises will take about 10 minutes to do and can be done daily.

CRUNCH

- Lie on your back with your knees bent
- Keep your hands on your thighs
- Reach up and slide your hands up and over the knees
- Make certain your lower back is totally off the ground
- Do ten repetitions

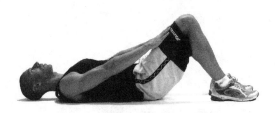

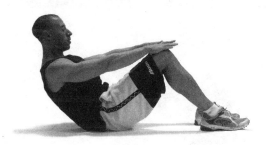

SINGLE LEG LIFT

- Lie on your back with your arms stretched straight over your head
- Bend one knee and keep the other straight on the ground
- Simultaneously lift your straight leg and your arms and touch your toes
- Make certain your lower back is totally off the ground
- Repeat with the other foot
- Do ten repetitions

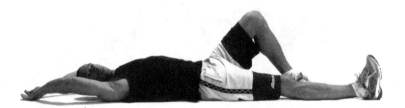

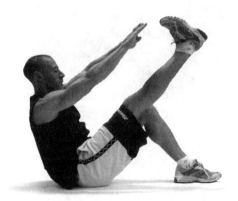

SIT UPS

- Lie on your back with your knees bent
- Keep your hands on your thighs and then slide them up over the knees and along the shins to the toes
- Do ten repetitions

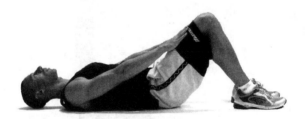

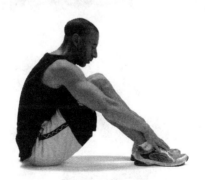

TOE TOUCH

- Lie on your back and extend both legs straight up above you
- Reach up and touch your toes, and if you can't touch your toes, go as far as you can, and work up to the toes over time
- Do ten repetitions

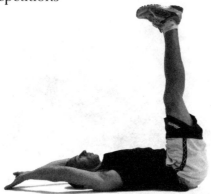

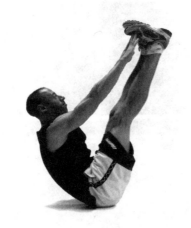

HEEL RAISE

- Lie on your back and extend both legs straight up above you
- Flex your toes back so your heels are pointing at the ceiling
- Put your arms straight along your body and keep your hands flat on the ground beside your hips
- Push your heels up raising your buttocks off the ground
- Do ten repetitions

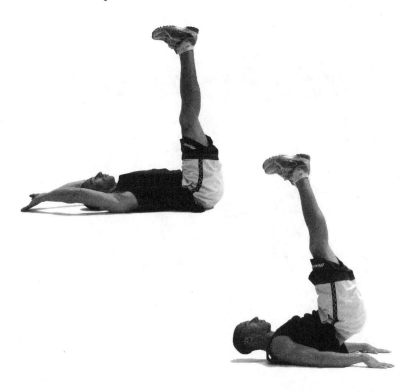

LEG STRETCH

- Lie on your back with your arms by your sides
- Lift your torso and one leg up, bending the knee and bringing it up to the chest
- Return to starting position
- Alternate legs
- Do ten repetitions

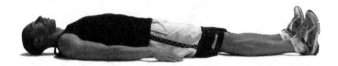

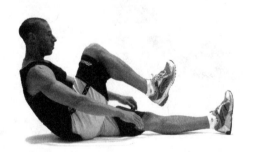

TWIST

- Lie on your back with your knees bent
- Cross the right foot over the left knee
- Put your left hand behind your head, and stretch your right arm straight out to the side
- Lift your torso, pushing off with your right hand, and touch your left elbow to the right knee. Make certain that the lower back is entirely off the ground.
- Do ten repetitions
- Switch sides and repeat

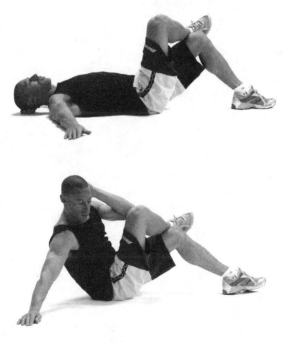

HOLD

- Lie on your back with your arms at your sides
- Cross your arms across your chest and lift up your torso about ten inches off the floor
- Hold this position for thirty seconds

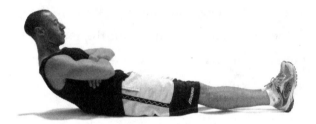

Core Exercises for Intermediates

Start your core exercises with the eight beginner core exercises, and then add the following six exercises.

The core exercises for intermediates may seem difficult at first. Never hold your breath while doing these exercises. If you are unable to do ten repetitions of each exercise at the beginning, do as many as you can and slowly work up to ten repetitions. Concentrate on maintaining the correct form when doing these exercises. It is more important to maintain the proper form than it is to complete all the repetitions. To get the most benefit from these exercises, remember to keep your toe flexed and to do slow repetitions. Do not rush through the repetitions. These exercises can be done daily.

If your fitness level improves to the point that you are no longer challenged by these exercises and wish to move to a more advanced level, consult a fitness instructor to get the proper exercises and techniques.

HANDSTAND WITH LEG LIFT

- Lie prone, facing the floor
- Lift your body up on your hands and toes
- Keep your body straight and rigid without lifting your buttocks
- Lift one leg up, keeping the leg straight and the toe flexed
- Do ten slow repetitions with this leg
- Switch legs and do ten slow repetitions with the other leg

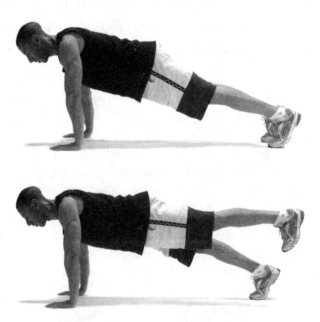

ELBOW STAND WITH LEG LIFT

- Lie prone, facing the floor
- Your elbows are under your shoulders and bent 90 degrees
- Raise your body up on your toes and distribute your weight evenly between your elbows and toes
- Keep your body straight and rigid and in a straight line without lifting your buttocks
- Lift one leg up, keeping the leg straight and the toe flexed
- Do ten slow repetitions with this leg
- Switch legs and do ten slow repetitions with the other leg

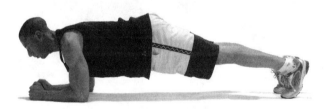

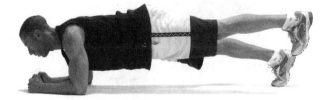

LATERAL HANDSTAND WITH LEG LIFT

- Lie on your side
- Push off the ground and distribute your weight between your hand and the side edge of your bottom foot
- Keep your torso straight and rigid, so your body is in a straight line
- Keeping your leg straight with your toe flexed and pointing down, slowly raise your upper leg
- Do ten repetitions then switch sides and legs

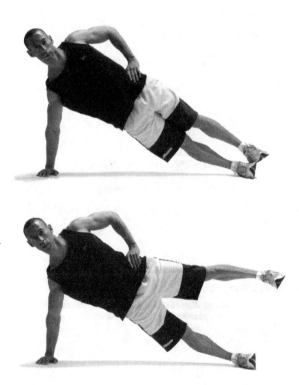

LATERAL ELBOW STAND WITH LEG LIFT

- Lie on your side with your forearm on the ground and your elbow under your shoulder
- Push up off your elbow creating a straight line from the ankle to the shoulder
- Only the elbow and the side edge of your bottom foot should be in contact with the ground
- Distribute your weight evenly between your elbow and the side of your foot
- Keep your torso straight and rigid, so your body is in a straight line and not sagging
- Keeping your leg straight with the toe flexed and pointing down, slowly raise the upper leg
- Do ten repetitions then switch sides and legs

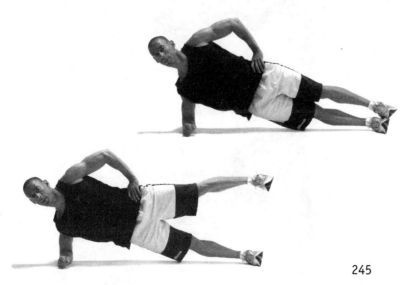

SUPINE HANDSTAND WITH LEG LIFT

- Lie face up
- Keeping your elbow under your shoulder, lift your body off the ground and distribute your weight evenly between your hands and heels
- Keep your torso straight and rigid and keep your buttocks up so your body is in a straight line
- Keeping your leg straight with your toe flexed up, slowly raise one leg and do ten repetitions
- Switch legs and do ten repetitions with the other leg

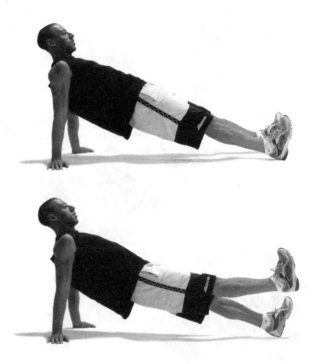

SUPINE ELBOW STAND WITH LEG LIFT

- Lie face up
- Keep your elbow under your shoulder and push off the ground distributing your weight evenly between the elbows and heels
- Keep your torso straight and rigid and keep your buttocks up, so your body is in a straight line
- Keeping your leg straight with your tow flexed, raise one leg for a slow count of ten repetitions
- Switch legs and do ten repetitions with the other leg

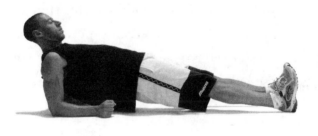

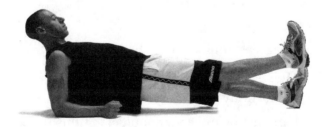

STRENGTH TRAINING

Strength training builds the muscle mass that is necessary to preserve strength, balance and functional ability. To maintain upper body strength, push-ups are one of the best exercises. To maintain lower body strength, squats are one of the best exercises.

Strength Training for Beginners

These exercises do not require you to purchase any special equipment and use only your body weight. They can be completed in about ten minutes. As no special equipment is required these exercises can be done even if you are traveling. These exercises can be done daily.

PUSH-UPS FOR UPPER BODY

- Stand two feet from a wall, extend your arms straight from your shoulders until you touch the wall
- Lower your body toward the wall, make sure your hands are just below your shoulders at this point

- Push away from the wall and return to the original position
- Do ten repetitions
- Work up to three sets of ten repetitions resting a minute between sets
- When you are able to do the wall push–ups, progress to doing push–ups off a counter top.
- Stand two feet from a counter top, extend your arms straight from the shoulders and rest your hands on the counter top
- Lower your body to the counter making sure your shoulders are directly above your hands
- Push away from the counter and return to the original position
- Do ten repetitions
- Work up to three sets of ten repetitions, resting a minute between sets

SQUATS FOR LOWER BODY

- Stand in front of a chair that has arms
- Stand with your feet hip–width apart

- Place your hands on the arms of the chair and lower yourself, pushing your buttocks behind you as if you will be sitting down in the chair
- When your buttocks almost touch the chair, pause, then slowly return to standing position
- Do three sets of ten repetitions with a one minute rest in between each set
- When you are comfortably able to do three sets of ten repetitions, then graduate to doing the same exercise without holding the arms of the chair
- When you are comfortably able to do three sets of ten repetitions of these, then try doing the same exercise with your arms folded over your chest

Strength Training for the Intermediate

Exercises that use only your body weight can be done daily. If you are adding extra weight by using dumbbells or if you are doing an increased amount of repetitions, then your muscles will need a day to recover, and you can do the exercise every other day.

PUSH-UPS FOR UPPER BODY

- Kneel on the floor with your hands on the floor directly below your shoulders and keep your arms straight
- Keep your stomach tight 'and lower your chest to the floor until it almost touches
- Raise yourself up to the original position
- When you are comfortably able to do three sets of ten repetitions of pushups from the kneeling position, then advance to doing the pushups from your toes
- Raise your body up on your toes and with your hands directly below your shoulders push up until your arms are fully extended
- Lower your body until your chest almost touches the floor
- Return to the starting position
- Do three sets of ten repetitions, resting a minute between sets

SQUATS FOR LOWER BODY

- Stand in front of a chair with no arms
- Males should hold 15-pound dumbbells in each hand, woman should hold 5-pound dumbbells in each hand

- Stand with your feet hip-width apart
- Slowly descend, pushing your buttocks behind you as if you will be sitting down in the chair
- When your buttocks almost touch the chair, pause, then slowly return to your starting position
- Do three sets of ten repetitions, resting a minute between sets

If you continue to do these intermediate lower and upper body strength training exercises, you will maintain your muscle tone.

You can do more advanced strength training exercises for even greater benefits. Consult a physical trainer for advice on the proper exercises and correct techniques. It is not wise to do more than forty-five minutes of strength training in one session. At this point, cortisol levels will increase and accelerate the aging process.

At a more advanced level of strength training, you should rest your muscles longer between training sessions. Muscles grow during the rest period following a workout. Depending on the intensity of the workout, muscles can take a few days to recover. Weight trainers require a more intense workout to challenge their muscles, thus requiring a longer time for recovery. Novices can work out every other day.

If you do join a gym and start training with weights, it may be more beneficial to train with free weights than with machines. A recent study done at Truman University found that lifting free weights expends more calories.

The study participants burned almost 50% more calories, doing two sets of ten squats while holding a weight than they did doing the same number of repetitions using a leg press machine with equivalent weight. The director of the Human Performance Lab at Truman University in Kirksville, Missouri, and coauthor of the study says the reason for this is, "with free weights, you activate more muscles for balance and control".

What Sabotages Exercise Routines?

- **Beginning an exercise program with enthusiasm and working out with high intensity for long periods of time resulting in pain or injury.** This requires a halt to our program while we recover, and often we fail to resume the exercises.

- **Not motivated enough to change old habits of inactivity.** Many times we begin an exercise program with good intentions but quickly determine we don't enjoy working out and quit. You may find it boring and tedious to do regular activity after being inactive for a long period of time. It usually takes us a few weeks to get used to change or a new regime in our lives. If you stick it out for a month, the increased activity makes you feel better and becomes more enjoyable and less of a chore.

- **Getting discouraged too quickly and falling off the "exercise wagon".** Expecting instant results is not reasonable. It took time to get out of shape and it will take time to get back into good physical condition. You might not see an instant weight loss or change in waist-line measurement, but if you don't get discouraged and continue the activity, in just a few months the results can be dramatic. When you start looking good and feeling strong, you will feel more confident and will want to continue. Being fit helps you to manage your daily activities, participate in your favorite sports and maintain a high quality of life well into your senior years.

- **Being too busy to exercise.** We all lead very active lives in modern society. Time is very valuable and the pressure is on us to get a lot done in a day. Investing time in yourself is one of the most important investments. Exercise gives you the energy and improved health to carry on with your many activities. An exercise program can impact every part of your life in a good way.

Part IV

INJURIES

CHAPTER 23

When Can Injuries Occur?

Anyone who participates in sports, whether professionally or recreationally is at risk of getting injured at some point in time. However, it is not only sporting activities that cause injuries. We are involved in activities in our everyday lives in which injuries can, and do occur. Gardening, spring cleaning, shoveling snow or playing with the grandchildren are all activities that can cause injury.

Even though sports and recreational activities can lead to injury, these activities are a great way to keep in shape and have fun while staying fit. If you are taking up a new sport, get proper instruction from the start. With proper technique, you will be less likely to get injured and more likely to appreciate the sport. Make certain you have the right equipment for the activity you are doing. Wear the proper shoes, elbow pads, helmet, mouth guard, etc. when required. If you do get injured, it is important to stop the activity that caused the injury and get medical attention before the injury worsens.

Many people who have not exercised or played sports for years return to activities without preparation. If you have lived a sedentary lifestyle, you must gradually improve your fitness level. If you rush back into an activity without proper conditioning, you will almost certainly experience aching muscles, strains, sprains and sometimes, more serious injury.

Start an exercise program slowly and allow the body to adapt. It is not wise to abruptly change the intensity and frequency of your workout. On occasion, we allow our fitness level to slip, and then try to get back into shape over a weekend. We might have a function to attend, such as a wedding or reunion, and want to look fabulous for this event. It is in these bursts of fitness mania that we can suffer injuries.

Sometimes injuries can take years to develop. There are about 150 joints in the human body that are protected by cartilage, and if this cartilage begins to degenerate because of trauma or overuse, secondary osteoarthritis can develop. Osteoarthritis is a chronic injury that can leave us in pain for the rest of our lives.

People may also have inherent characteristics that predispose them to certain injuries. High arches, flat feet, different leg lengths, abnormal kneecap position or a family history of arthritis, are just a few.

Even though we might take all the necessary precautions, injuries can still happen. I will discuss some of the more common injuries that can occur, the causes and the recommended treatments.

Rehabilitation Exercises

Many injuries require a series of exercises for rehabilitation. It is recommended to have a qualified physician or a physiotherapist design the exercise program specific to your injury and instruct you on the correct way to do these exercises. More harm than good can be done if the proper exercise or the proper form of doing the exercise is not followed.

CHAPTER 24

Knee Injuries

The knee joint is made up of bones, cartilage, muscles, tendons and ligaments all working together to provide flexibility and stability, allowing our legs to bend, swivel and straighten.

The three bones in the knee joint are the femur (thighbone), the tibia (shinbone) and the patella (kneecap). The ends of the femur and tibia are covered with articular cartilage. This acts as a cushion to prevent the femur and tibia from grinding against each other. On the top of the tibia, there are extra pads of cartilage called menisci. Each knee has two menisci, the medial (inside) meniscus and the lateral (outside) meniscus.

The quadriceps is the large muscle in the front of the thigh that helps straighten the knee. The hamstring is the muscle located at the back of the thigh which helps bend the knee.

The tendons in the knee are the quadriceps tendon and the patellar tendon. The quadriceps tendon connects to the top of the patella. The patellar tendon connects to the bottom of the patella and attaches to the top of the tibia.

There are four ligaments in the knee that connect the femur to the tibia and keep the leg stable. These are:

- The medial collateral ligament which connects the femur to the tibia along the inside of the knee. It helps keep the inner part of the knee stable, and controls the sideways motion of the knee and keeps it from bending inward.

- The lateral collateral ligament connects the femur to the tibia along the outside of the knee. It helps keep the outer part of the knee stable and keeps it from bending outward.

- The anterior cruciate ligament connects the femur to the tibia at the center of the knee. It controls forward motion and rotation and keeps the tibia from sliding out in front of the femur.

- The posterior cruciate ligament connects the femur to the tibia at the back of the knee. It controls backward motion and keeps the tibia from sliding out under the femur.

I will describe a few of the more common knee injuries.

Anatomy of the Knee

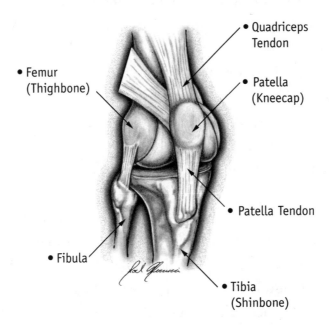

• Quadriceps
  Tendon

• Femur
  (Thighbone)

• Patella
  (Kneecap)

• Patella Tendon

• Fibula

• Tibia
  (Shinbone)

PATELLOFEMORAL SYNDROME

Patellofemoral syndrome (PFS) is one of the most common causes of knee pain. It is an injury that occurs between the patella and the femur. It can occur in two ways, either by misalignment of the kneecap or by repetitive overuse.

The patella (kneecap) is a bone that lies in a groove in the front of the femur (the thighbone). PFS usually causes pain in the inner knee area or behind the knee, and is aggravated by running, jumping, climbing stairs, descending stairs, squatting or prolonged sitting with the knees in a bent position.

Magnetic resonance imaging (MRI) can confirm the diagnosis.

What causes it?

- Misalignment of the kneecap. Normally, the patella is pulled up over the thighbone in a straight line by the thigh muscles (quadriceps). In PFS, the kneecap tracks toward the outer side of the thighbone. This misalignment causes the underside of the kneecap to abrade, resulting in inflammation and pain.
- Overuse and overloading the knee joint. Excessive exercise can cause microtrauma in the area of the patellofemoral joint. This results in irritation and inflammation of the kneecap.

What are the symptoms?

- Pain in the inner knee area or behind the knee.
- Pain is experienced after prolonged sitting. This is called the "theater" or "movie sign" symptom. If the knee is more severely injured, the pain will occur more quickly than if the knee is not as badly inflamed. In the sitting position, when the knee is bent at right angles, the knee joint is in the highest degree of compression and will cause pain if it is inflamed.
- Pain is experienced while ascending or descending stairs or when squatting. These actions put the knee under a high degree of compression.

What is the treatment?

- Reduce pain and inflammation by icing and taking anti-inflammatory medication.
- Stop the activity that originally injured the knee.
- Avoid knee movements that cause pain.
- Daily exercises are essential. Consult with a physician to have your injury assessed. An exercise program should be designed for your specific needs, and proper instruction given to you for doing these exercises.

A common belief is that a weakness in the inner portion of the quadriceps muscle causes the patella to be pulled out of position. However, PFS exists in athletes and people who have well developed inner quadriceps muscles. In these cases, when the pain persisted, some medical professionals believed that lateral release surgery should be used to treat the problem.

This operation consists of cutting the lateral stabilizing ligament of the patella. I believe this procedure is barbaric and should be banned. PFS can be treated with more conservative treatments in every situation.

I developed a test that can measure the electrical contractions of the leg muscles. Electromyography (EMG) is an existing test that is done to assess the health of a muscle and the nerves controlling the muscle. In this test, a needle electrode is inserted through the skin into the muscle and the electrical activity detected by this electrode is displayed on a monitor. The muscle is contracted and information is collected on the ability of the muscle to respond when the nerves are stimulated.

I modified the Electromyography (EMG) test in such a way that the electrical contractions of the muscles can be measured. I found that it's not the strength of the inside quadriceps muscle that causes the patella to be misaligned, but the timing of the contraction of the muscle. A person prone to PFS has the inside muscle contracting a millisecond later than the outside muscle.

Using the EMG technique, with a modification to the electrode, we can observe the electrical contraction of the inside and outside muscles. In this test, the electrode is attached onto the surface of the skin above the muscles to be tested. You are asked to contract the muscles several times and the results are plotted on a graph. The muscle contractions can be observed to determine whether the inside muscle is contracting later than the outside muscle.

If this is the case, the inside muscle can be taught through biofeedback techniques to contract earlier and thereby straighten the path taken by the kneecap against the thighbone. Biofeedback technique is used to help people improve their own health by using signals from their body.

With the electrodes still connected to the muscles, you are asked to do specific exercises and observe on the graph which exercise will cause the inside muscle to contract at the same time or sooner than the outside muscle. Each person will be different and will require exercises specific to them. Once these are determined, you can practise these exercises and train the inside muscle to contract sooner than the outside muscle. The EMG test should be repeated in a month or two to see if progress has been made.

Improper Firing of Muscles

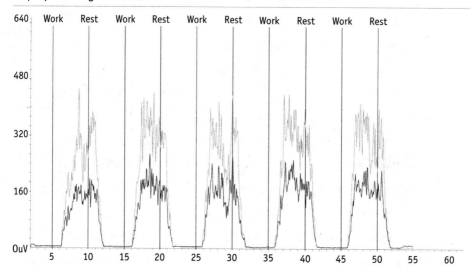

Proper Firing of Muscles

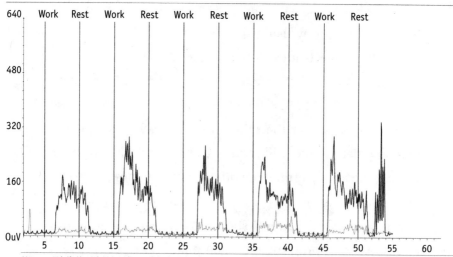

Vastus Medialis (Inside) Muscle is in black
Vastus Lateralis (Outside) Muscle is in gray

CHONDROMALACIA PATELLA

Chondromalacia is the softening and eventual degeneration of the cartilage behind the kneecap and in the groove in which it tracks. Abnormal tracking of the kneecap causes the cartilage to wear down.

Chondromalacia that occurs in adolescents or young adults is usually caused by overuse or trauma. It occurs more often in females than in males, and many of the affected adolescents have abnormal alignment of the kneecaps.

In older adults, the cartilage breaks down as a result of the normal aging process. This is one of the first places in the body that cartilage breaks down. This process gradually progresses, and eventually leads to osteoarthritis of the knee.

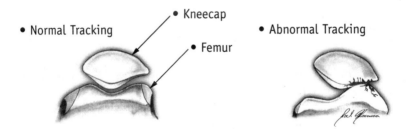

Magnetic resonance imaging (MRI) can be used to confirm the diagnosis.

What causes it?

- Overuse
- Trauma to the knee
- Misalignment of the kneecap
- Aging

What are the symptoms?

- Pain in the front of the knee that worsens when climbing or descending stairs or when walking uphill
- Pain when squatting, kneeling or when sitting with the knee bent for a long period of time
- A grating sensation when the knee is extended

What is the Treatment?

- Take anti-inflammatory medication to relieve the pain and swelling.
- Avoid activities that cause the pain.
- Exercise to strengthen the quadriceps and hamstrings. Consult with a physician for the proper exercises and techniques.

- A stabilizing brace may be recommended for the knee.
- Physiotherapy which may include electrical stimulation to strengthen the muscles.
- If all other methods fail, surgery could be an option. Fragments of damaged cartilage are removed using arthroscopic surgery.

PATELLAR/QUADRICEPS TENDONITIS

Often referred to as "jumper's knee", this condition usually affects people who are participating in sports or activities where jumping is involved. The condition is seen in those who participate in activities such as basketball, tennis, distance running, mountain climbing, ballet or high-impact aerobics.

Tendons attach muscles to bone. In the knee, the quadriceps is connected to the patella by the quadriceps tendon, and the patellar tendon connects the patella (kneecap) to the tibia (shinbone). Patellar tendonitis is an inflammation of the patellar tendon, and quadriceps tendonitis is an inflammation of the quadriceps tendon. Inflammation is caused by overuse and repetitive stress on the knee. Under these conditions, the tendons begin to degenerate and weaken. If not rested, they become more susceptible to injury.

271

X-rays, ultra sound and magnetic resonance imaging (MRI) can confirm the injury and reveal the areas of tear in the tendon.

What causes it?

- Overuse. Overuse injuries occur when you repeat a specific activity until microtears of the tendon tissue appear. These tears cause inflammation, pain and swelling. Any sport which involves running or jumping can cause this injury.
- Tight leg muscles. Reduced flexibility of the hamstring and quadriceps muscles can increase the strain on tendons.
- Muscular imbalance. If some muscles in the legs are much stronger than others, they can over stress the tendons. This uneven tension can cause tendonitis.
- A raised kneecap. If the patella sits higher on the knee joint than normal, increased strain on the patellar tendon can occur.
- Leg misalignment. The leg bones can be misaligned slightly, putting strain on the tendons.
- Ankles rolling inwards (overpronating) during walking or running.

What are the symptoms?

- Pain is localized in the front of the knees, just under the kneecap, and will appear after sports or recreational activities.
- Pain can be severe when landing a jump or running.
- Pain will increase when walking or running down stairs or when rising from a sitting position.
- A feeling of weakness in the knee and swelling just under the kneecap. Although, the swelling is usually not significant.

What is the treatment?

- Ice the knee after exercise to reduce swelling and inflammation.
- Take anti–inflammatory medication to relieve the pain and inflammation.
- Stop the activity that causes pain and rest the knee. Initially, pain may appear early in the workout, ease up, and again become worse at the end of the workout. If you continue to exercise with the pain, you will be able to perform at a normal level at first. However, if you continue to work through the pain, without resting

the injury, the pain will become persistent during and after the activity. Permanent damage, such as calcification, can be done to the tendon.

- Keep the knee straight when sitting and avoid squatting.
- Exercise to strengthen the quadriceps. Consult with a physician or physiotherapist to get the proper exercises and instruction on how to do them.
- Avoid sports that require jumping, such as basketball, tennis, football and volleyball. Avoid squats, stair-steppers and lunges. Swimming, walking and cross-country skiing can be done as aerobic activities.
- Stretching hip flexors, quadriceps, hamstrings and lateral muscle groups is essential. Consult with a physician or physiotherapist to get the proper stretches and instruction on how to do them.
- Wearing an infra-patellar strap or knee brace during exercise could help.
- Orthotics to reduce overpronation.
- Warm up before exercise to prevent reinjury of the knee.
- There has been some reported success with aprotinin, pentosan and polysulphate injections. At present, The Institute of Sport Medicine & Wellness Centre in Toronto is the only medical center using pentosan and polysulphate for this application.

Cortisone, a powerful anti-inflammatory drug, is often injected into the tendon to make it less painful and swollen. The problem with cortisone is that the effect of the cortisone injection often wears off quickly, and there is a risk of tendon rupture after the injection.

Aprotinin is not a steroid or cortisone. It is a protein that is obtained, and purified from cows' lungs. It has been used in medicine as a drug in heart surgery for many years, and only recently it has been found effective in treating chronic tendon injuries.

Aprotinin inhibits enzymes in the body that break down protein, including tendon protein. Therefore, it might be able to reverse some of the tendon damage seen in tendonitis. It is also less likely to rupture a tendon than a cortisone injection. However, be aware that some people might have an allergic reaction to this drug.

ILIOTIBIAL BAND SYNDROME

The iliotibial band (ITB) is a thickened portion of connective tissue that runs down the outside of the thigh, from the hip all the way down the side of the thigh to just below the knee. The tension and movement of this band can be altered by the various muscles that it is attached to. At the top, there is the gluteus maximus muscle attaching from the back and the tensor fascia latae muscle attaching from the front. Near the bottom of the ITB, the outer portion of the quadriceps and the outer portion of the hamstrings have some insertion points as well.

If the ITB is pulled tight by one of the muscles mentioned above, it can be pulled out of balance and this leads to ITB syndrome. Running up and down hills can sometimes trigger ITB syndrome because this action uses more of the gluteus maximus muscle than running on flat ground and this causes a shift in the ITB.

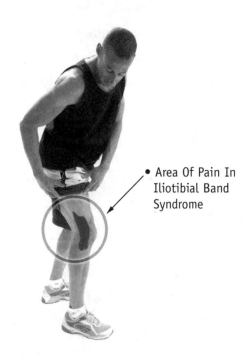

• Area Of Pain In Iliotibial Band Syndrome

The inflammation could be in the iliotibial band itself or in the bursa. Bursae are fluid filled sacs that lubricate areas where friction occurs. If the ITB is pulled tight, it can put pressure on the bursa and this can cause the bursa to become inflamed and painful. Both of these conditions will result in ITB syndrome and pain to the lateral (outside) part of the knee.

Magnetic resonance imaging (MRI) can be used to confirm the injury.

What causes it?

- Running on a slanted surface or uneven roads can irritate the lower portion of the ITB and cause it to become inflamed.
- Running up and down hills or stairs can irritate the ITB because of the change in motion of the hip and knee and the tension of the gluteus maximus muscle.
- Overpronation of the foot causes the tibia to turn inwards which will pull the ITB forward and under the inside of the knee causing irritation.
- Uneven leg length can cause an imbalance and put more pressure on the ITB.

- Muscle imbalances can pull the ITB out of position and cause irritation.

What are the symptoms?

- Lateral (outside) knee pain
- Pain is worse, if running up and down hills or climbing stairs
- May experience pain in the outside of the thigh
- Pain may not occur until half way into a run
- Pain could be severe

What is the treatment?

- Icing will help with redness, swelling and pain.
- Take anti–inflammatory medication to relieve pain and swelling.
- Avoid the activity that caused the injury. Swimming could be used as a cardiovascular activity if the injury is not severe or once the pain is under control.
- Gentle stretching can be done. The quadriceps, hamstrings and gluteus maximus as well as the ITB

can be stretched gently. It would be wise to be assessed by a professional to determine which muscles need to be worked on and balanced, as each individual will have different needs.

- Ultrasound can be used to control inflammation and assist healing.
- Changing footwear may be essential to keep the injury from reoccurring. Motion-control shoes and orthotics may be required to keep the foot from overpronating.
- Stay on flat roads. Avoid excessive hill running and cambered roads.
- Strengthen quadriceps, hamstrings and calf muscles. Consult with a physician or physiotherapist for exercises and proper techniques.
- Recovery is between three to six weeks.

MENISCUS TEAR

The knee joint is made up of three bones, the femur (thigh bone), the tibia (shinbone) and the patella (kneecap). There are two menisci in each knee that rest between the thighbone and the shin bone. These are made of tough cartilage and are C-shaped with a wedged profile. One is the medial meniscus, and the other is the lateral meniscus. Their purpose is to help keep the knee stabilized and provide cushioning between the shinbone and the thighbone allowing these bones to glide smoothly against each other without damage.

The outer part of the meniscus is nourished by small blood vessels. The inner part has a limited blood supply. If damage is done to the outer part of the meniscus, it will often fully heal because there is a supply of blood vessels to this area. If damage is done to the inner part of the meniscus, where there is a limited blood supply, then the damage will be less likely to heal.

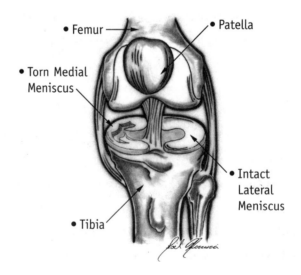

X-ray and magnetic resonance imaging (MRI) can be used to confirm the diagnosis.

What causes it?

- Twisting or rotational stress to the knee, such as aggressive pivoting or sudden stops and turns
- Trauma to the knee
- In older adults, meniscus tear can occur from degenerative changes to the knee

What are the symptoms?

- Mild to moderate swelling of the knee
- Knee pain, which can be localized to the side of the knee the tear is on
- Limited motion of the knee joint
- Mechanical complaints, such as locking of the knee, clicking or a feeling of giving way
- Collection of water on the knee

What is the treatment?

- Rest, icing and elevation along with anti-inflammatory medication may correct the problem, if not too serious. Blood vessels feed the outer edges of the meniscus, therefore small tears on the outer edges can heal on their own.
- Physiotherapy and strengthening exercises. Consult with a physician or physiotherapist for the proper exercises and techniques.
- If the meniscus tear physically interferes with knee movement, it may have to be repaired or partially removed using arthroscopic surgery.

OSTEOARTHRITIS OF THE KNEE

Osteoarthritis is the most common type of arthritis of the knee. It usually occurs in middle age or older adults. It is a slowly progressive degenerative disease in which the joint cartilage gradually wears away.

X-rays and magnetic resonance imaging (MRI) can diagnose this disease.

What are the symptoms?

- The knee is stiff and swollen and is difficult to bend or straighten
- Pain is usually worse in the morning then lessens after moving about
- Pain can increase with walking, climbing stairs or kneeling
- There could be a deformity of the knee, like bow–legedness

What is the treatment?

- Anti–inflammatory medication to reduce pain and swelling
- Physiotherapy and exercise to strengthen the knee and restore joint movement. Consult with a physician or physiotherapist to obtain the proper exercises and techniques.
- Glucosamine can sometimes relieve symptoms
- Arthroscopic surgery can clear the debris, or repair a torn cartilage
- A partial or total knee replacement

- Cartilage grafting is sometimes possible
- Cartilage regeneration and transplant. There has been some work done with regenerative cartilage injections. Growth hormone and various nutrients are injected directly into the knee to provide relief from pain.
- Injection of hyaluronic acid into arthritic joints. Hyaluronic acid is able to hold more water than any other natural substance, therefore it plays an important role in lubricating the joint.

CHAPTER 25

Foot and Ankle Injuries

FLAT FEET

Flat feet or pes planus is a condition where the foot has a flattened arch. The inner side of the human foot is meant to have an arch or gap between the foot and the ground. With flat feet or fallen arches, the entire sole of the foot is flat against the ground. We are all born with flat feet, but by the age of about ten, the tendons that attach to the bone of the foot become stronger and tighten, forming an arch. In most people, a low arch or flat foot will cause no problems and will require no treatment.

What causes it?

- Can be hereditary
- Obesity
- A ruptured or weakened tendon
- Abnormal walking pattern where the foot overpronates (rolls in too much)
- Conditions such as cerebral palsy or muscular dystrophy can lead to flat feet

What are the symptoms?

- Many people do not experience symptoms
- May experience corns and hard skin under the soles of the foot
- Uneven shoe wear pattern
- Arch area may be painful
- May experience calf, knee and hip pain

What is the treatment?

- Use of orthotics to take pressure away from the arch
- Footwear with motion control

- Anti–inflammatory medication to reduce pain and swelling

HIGH ARCH FEET

High arch or pes cavus is an excessively elevated arch in the foot. Highly arched feet are less common than flat feet and tend to be more painful due to the stresses placed on the section of the foot between the ankle and the toes (mid foot).

What causes it?

- May be hereditary
- Underlying neurological problem

What are the symptoms?

- Foot pain when walking, standing or running
- Usually accompanied by crooked toes called hammertoes
- Foot may roll outward slightly which is opposite of a pronated foot

- May have corns and calluses under the bases of the first and fifth toe
- May have difficulty fitting shoes because of the high arch and clawed toes
- Foot will be stiffer and less mobile

What is the treatment?

- Orthotics can be worn
- Pads can be worn to take the pressure off painful areas
- Surgery to flatten the foot may sometimes be necessary

BUNIONS

A bunion is an abnormal bony bump that forms at the base of the big toe after this joint is stressed for a long period of time. The base of the big toe, or metatarsophalangeal joint, can continue to get larger and more painful. The bigger the bunion gets, the more painful it will be, and the more difficult it will be to walk. The big toe may angle toward the second toe, forcing it out of alignment and deforming the foot. Nine out of ten bunions occur in women, and the cause is usually from wearing tight shoes and high heels.

What causes it?

- Can be hereditary
- Caused mostly by wearing tight narrow shoes and high heels
- Can be a result of arthritis that affects the big toe joint

What are the symptoms?

- Pain, redness and swelling at the base of the big toe
- Large bony bump at the base of the big toe
- Can result in the big toe leaning towards the second toe, and actually pushing it under or over the second toe, causing deformity

What is the treatment?

- Avoid shoes that are tight, narrow and have high heels
- Wear shoes that do not put pressure on the bunion
- Wear protective pads to cushion the painful area
- Surgery might be required to realign the bones, ligaments and tendons, and bring the big toe back to the proper position. A long recovery period is common.

ACHILLES TENDONITIS

The Achilles tendon is the largest tendon in the human body. It is the tendon that connects the muscles of the calf to the heel. Achilles tendonitis is an inflammation of the Achilles tendon.

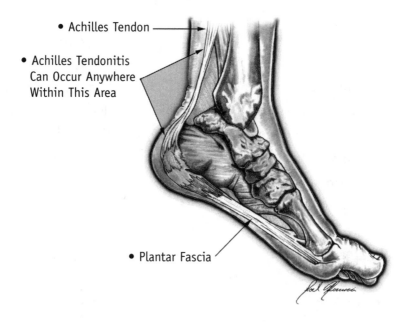

- Achilles Tendon
- Achilles Tendonitis Can Occur Anywhere Within This Area
- Plantar Fascia

Magnetic resonance imaging (MRI) can detect inflammation in the Achilles tendon.

What causes it?

- Overuse injuries. These are most commonly seen in younger individuals or athletes participating in sports that require jumping, such as basketball. Jumping puts stress on the Achilles tendon.
- Arthritis can cause bony growths in the area of the Achilles tendon causing the tendon to become inflamed. Tendonitis due to arthritic spurs is more common in middle aged and older individuals.
- Trauma

What are the symptoms?

- Pain in the heel area when walking or running
- Tendon is painful to the touch and may be swollen
- Pain in the tendon area when you stand on your toes

What is the treatment?

- Anti-inflammatory medication
- Physiotherapy to stretch the muscle and tendon, and to strengthen the calf muscle. Consult with a

physician or physiotherapist for proper exercises
and techniques.

- Stop the activity that caused the problem or any
  activity that causes pain
- Braces or boots can be used to limit ankle motion
- Ultrasound treatment
- Surgery may be required to remove inflamed tissue or
  any part of the tendon that has become abnormal
- There has been some reported success with aprotinin
  injections

Aprotinin is not a steroid or cortisone. It is a protein that
is obtained and purified from cows' lungs. For many years,
it has been used in medicine as a drug in heart surgery.
Recently, it has been found to be effective in treating chronic
tendon injuries.

Aprotinin inhibits enzymes in the body that break
down protein, including tendon protein. Therefore, it might
be able to reverse some of the tendon damage seen in
tendonitis. It is also less likely to rupture a tendon than a
cortisone injection.

Cortisone is a powerful anti-inflammatory drug that is
injected into the tendon in order to make it less painful and
swollen. The problem is that the effect of the cortisone injection often wears off quickly, and there is risk of tendon

rupture after the injection. This is especially serious with the Achilles tendon, since there are no other tendons nearby to take the pressure if it snaps. Be aware that some people might have an allergic reaction to aprotinin.

SPRAINED ANKLE

A sprained ankle is a very common injury. Ankle ligaments are elastic structures that hold the ankle bone and joint in position. They protect the ankle joint during twisting and turning motions. Ligaments will stretch within their limits, and then return to their normal position. If the ligaments are pushed beyond their normal limits, a sprain will occur.

An X-ray should be taken to insure that the bone has not been broken. Magnetic resonance imaging (MRI) will show the extent of the injury to the ligaments.

What causes it?

- A sprain occurs if the foot twists or turns beyond its normal limits.
  A Grade 1 sprain is a slight stretching with some damage to the ligament.

A Grade 2 sprain is when there is partial tearing of the ligament.

A Grade 3 sprain is when there is a complete tear of the ligament.

What are the symptoms?

- Pain and swelling in the ankle area. Pain will depend on the amount of damage that has been done to the ligament.
- When the ligament has been completely torn, there will be instability in the ankle joint.

What is the treatment?

- Ice should be applied immediately to reduce the swelling. The ankle should be iced for 20 to 30 minutes, three times daily.
- Take anti-inflammatory medication to reduce pain and swelling.
- For the first 24 to 48 hours, rest the ankle, and do not put weight on the ankle.

- Elevate the ankle to reduce swelling.
- Use compression bandages to immobilize, and support the ankle.
- If the ankle does not respond to rest, ice, compression and elevation, it would be advisable to consult with a physician. Frequently, with Grade 2 sprains, a brace is recommended to provide ankle stabilization while the ligaments heal. Do not force the ankle to move, or put weight on it, if you experience pain.
- Grade 3 sprains require immobilization. A short leg cast or leg brace can be used for 2 to 3 weeks. Surgery is rarely required.
- Ultrasound treatments may be used to reduce the pain and swelling.
- Physiotherapy to increase the range of motion and flexibility and to strengthen the ankle. Consult with a physiotherapist for proper exercises and techniques.

PLANTAR FASCIITIS

Plantar fasciitis is a common painful foot condition. It is an inflammation of the band of tissue (plantar fascia) that runs from the heel along the arch to the ball of the foot. It can be found in all age groups, but is most common in middle aged men and women. Plantar fasciitis is a common problem among people active in sports, especially running.

Ultrasound can be used to confirm the diagnosis. The fascia normally measures 2 to 4 millimeters. A measurement of 4.5 millimeters or above would indicate this condition.

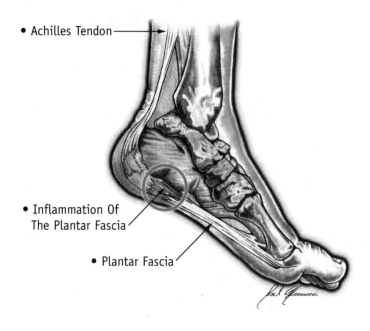

- Achilles Tendon

- Inflammation Of The Plantar Fascia

- Plantar Fascia

What causes it?

- Rapid change in activity level
- Being active in sports, such as running or aerobics

- Being overweight
- Being pregnant
- Can be hereditary
- Aging – as the arch of the foot begins to sag, it puts stress on the plantar fascia
- Running on soft surfaces, such as sand
- Running on hills
- Having flat feet or high arched feet can put you at risk
- Wearing shoes with poor arch support or stiff soles

What are the symptoms?

- Sharp pain in the inside part of the bottom of the heel
- More severe pain with the first steps in the morning
- Pain after prolonged standing or walking
- Pain at the beginning of a sports activity that lessens during activity
- Mild swelling in the heel area

What is the treatment?

- Icing and taking anti-inflammatory medication for pain.

- Physical therapy to stretch the plantar fascia and Achilles tendon and to strengthen the lower leg muscles which stabilize the heel. Consult with a physiotherapist for the proper exercises and techniques.
- Stop doing the activity that caused the problem.
- Orthotics can be worn.
- Cortisone injections may be used with caution. Cortisone may cause shrinking of the natural fat pad under the heel.
- Lose weight if you are overweight, especially if you are a woman. Obesity is present in 90% of the women with plantar fasciitis and in 40% of the men with this injury.
- Surgery may be required in some cases as a last resort. A small incision is made on the inside of the heel and the inflamed tissue is released or removed.
- Extracorporeal shock wave treatment has been shown to be successful.

Shock wave treatment delivers pulses of energy in the form of 1,500 to 2,000 sonic waves, into the painful area over a period of about ten minutes. Pain relief is usually immediate. This treatment should not be used on children, pregnant women or people who have a history of bleeding problems.

OSTEOARTHRITIS OR DEGENERATIVE ARTHRITIS OF THE FOOT AND ANKLE

The foot consists of 28 bones and more than 30 joints. Ligaments, which are tough bands of tissue, hold the bones and joints in place. Arthritis can develop in one or more of these joints.

X-ray, computed tomography (CT) or magnetic resonance imaging (MRI) can be used to diagnose and evaluate this condition.

What causes it?

- Arthritis develops with age. The thin covering over the ends of the bone, called the cartilage, begins to wear and tear after years of use. This results in pain, inflammation and swelling in the joint. A past injury to a joint can also cause arthritis to develop. This is sometimes referred to as traumatic arthritis, and can occur several months or years after the initial injury.

What are the symptoms?

- Pain

- Swelling
- Reduced motion
- Difficulty walking

What is the treatment?

- Anti-inflammatory drugs to reduce swelling and pain
- Physiotherapy and exercise. Consult with a physician or physiotherapist for the proper exercise program and instruction.
- Controlling your weight
- Using an arch support in your shoes
- Using a brace or cane as an aid when walking
- Steroid injection into the affected joint
- Arthroscopic surgery may be required to remove bone spurs or debris in the joint. In this procedure a small camera is inserted into the joint allowing the surgeon to assess the problem. Tiny shavers, knives and forceps are used to clean the joint area.
- Fusion surgery can be performed. This surgery eliminates the joint completely by welding the bones together. Pins and plates are used to hold the bones together until they heal. This surgery has a high success rate.

- Joint replacement can be performed, but ankle joint replacement is not as successful as hip or knee replacement. The implant may loosen or fail requiring more surgery.

- There has been some work done with regenerative cartilage injections. To provide relief from pain, growth hormone and various nutrients are injected directly into the arthritic joint. Some experimental work has been done with injection of hyaluronic acid into arthritic joints. Hyaluronic acid is able to hold more water than any other natural substance, thus it plays an important role in lubricating the joint. Hyaluronic acid is used in cosmetic surgery to fill in wrinkles. The hyaluronic acid used for arthritis has a higher molecular weight than that used for cosmetic surgery.

CHAPTER 26

Elbow Injuries

OVERUSE SYNDROME

Tennis elbow and golfer's elbow are examples of overuse syndrome of the elbow, sometimes known as repetitive strain injury or cumulative trauma disorder.

TENNIS ELBOW

Tennis elbow is the most common elbow injury. It affects an equal number of men and women and most patients are in the 35 to 65 year old age group. Anyone who repetitively stresses their wrist, such as plumbers, painters or gardeners, or people who play sports such as racquet sports, fencing or golf, are at risk of developing tennis elbow.

An X–ray will rule out a fracture or arthritis. More comprehensive imaging, such as magnetic resonance imaging (MRI) is rarely done.

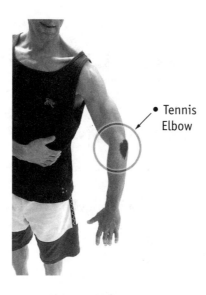

• Tennis Elbow

What causes it?

■ Repeated contractions of the forehand muscles that are used to straighten and raise the hand and wrist

- Small tears develop in the tendon that attaches the muscles of the forearm to the arm bone at the elbow joint

What are the symptoms?

- Pain on the outside of the elbow that is worsened by cocking the wrist back or grasping objects
- Pain radiating down the forearm
- Inability to straighten or flex the arm
- Swelling at the elbow

What is the treatment?

- Anti–inflammatory medication
- Ice the injury
- Use an elbow brace during activities
- Correct your technique. When playing sports, rackets should be the proper size and have the proper grip. An instructor should be consulted to evaluate your swing, and to determine if you are hitting the ball in the proper position.

- Analyze the way you use your arm while doing tasks to determine the best way to reduce stress on the injured arm.
- Cortisone injections
- Exercises to strengthen the muscles and tendons. Consult a physician or a physical therapist for required exercises and techniques.
- Usually, surgery is not necessary for tennis elbow. In extreme cases, a portion of the damaged tendon can be removed, or the attachment of the tendon can be released.
- Extracorpeal shock wave treatment has been shown to be successful

Shock wave treatment delivers pulses of energy, in the form of 1,500 to 2,000 sonic waves into the painful area over a period of about ten minutes. In most cases, pain relief is immediate.

On average, two to three treatments are needed over a three week period. Clinical experience from seven countries around the world has shown a 70% success rate in the reduction of pain. In many cases, results from the first treatment are so dramatic that patients feel that a second treatment is not necessary.

I have used extracorpeal shock wave treatment in over 2,500 cases, and have found a 90% success rate. I encourage my patients to have at least two treatments, even if they are feeling better after the first.

GOLFER'S ELBOW

Golfer's elbow is a similar injury to tennis elbow. It is an over-use injury, and both are forms of tendonitis. Usually, the pain in golfer's elbow is on the inside of the elbow, and can

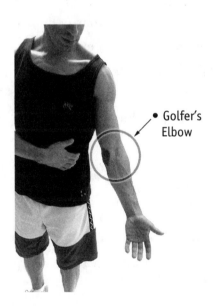

• Golfer's
Elbow

radiate down the forearm when picking up objects. Most patients are men in the 20 to 50 year old age group, but the injury can happen to anyone who repetitively stresses the wrists or fingers. This injury is seen in many athletes, not just golfers.

An X-ray will rule out a fracture or arthritis. More comprehensive imaging, such as magnetic resonance imaging (MRI), is rarely done.

What causes it?

- Repetitive use activity, such as golf, racket sports, carpentry, painting, raking, etc. Damage is done to the muscles and tendons that control the wrist and fingers.
- Sudden force to the elbow or wrist

What are the symptoms?

- Pain on the inside of the elbow
- Pain radiating down the forearm when picking up objects

What is the treatment?

- Rest the arm and stop doing the activity that caused the injury
- Anti-inflammatory medication
- Ice the injury
- Exercises to strengthen and stretch the muscles and tendon. Consult a physician or physiotherapist for correct exercises and techniques.
- Cortisone injections
- Extracorpeal shock wave treatment, as recommended in tennis elbow, may not work with this injury because of the proximity of the ulnar nerve. This treatment can cause damage to the nerve.

CHAPTER 27

Wrist Injuries

CARPAL TUNNEL

Carpal tunnel syndrome (CTS) is an inflammation of the wrist due to repetitive motion. The carpal tunnel is a small tunnel, located on the palm side of the wrist, formed by the wrist bones and ligaments. The median nerve and several tendons pass through the carpal tunnel from the forearm to the hand. Carpal tunnel syndrome is caused by activities that put pressure on the median nerve, and decrease its blood supply, leading to numbness, pain, tingling and weakness in the wrist and fingers. Women are three times as likely to develop CTS as men. In women, the incidence of CTS increases after menopause, and in men, during middle age.

What Causes It?

- Repetitive motions that involve only part of the hand, such as the fingers. Activities, such as typing, knitting, playing an instrument can cause CTS.
- Wrist injuries
- Pregnancy – CTS occurs in 28% of pregnant women
- Hormone imbalance, such as menopause
- Smoking and obesity can increase the chances of getting CTS
- Conditions such as diabetes, hypothyroidism and rheumatoid arthritis

What Are the Symptoms?

- Tingling, numbness or weakness in the hand or fingers, especially the thumb, index and middle fingers
- Decreased grip strength and sense of weakness in the hands
- Pain can radiate from the wrist up the arm to the shoulder, or radiate down from the wrist to the fingers
- Pain worsens at night

What Is the Treatment?

- Stop doing the activity that caused the problem and rest the hand.
- Change the way you do the activity. Rest more often, change the position of the hand, improve your posture and don't do the activity as long or as often.
- Use a wrist brace
- Stretch and strengthen your hands and arms. Consult with your doctor or physiotherapist to get the proper exercises and techniques.
- Surgery is usually not necessary, but can be done in extreme cases. The ligament that forms the roof of the carpal tunnel is cut to make more room in the tunnel and relieve the pressure on the median nerve.
- If the injury is caused by typing, a more ergonomically designed keyboard and work area may help.
- If CTS is induced by pregnancy, then splinting the wrist in a neutral position may reduce pressure on the carpal tunnel. In pregnant women this condition usually clears up after the baby is born and doesn't occur again unless there is another pregnancy.

ARTHRITIS OF THE WRIST

Although there are many kinds of arthritis, most wrist pain is caused by only two, osteoarthritis and rheumatoid arthritis.

Osteoarthritis damages the articular cartilage that covers the ends of the bone. The bones rub against each other causing pain, swelling, stiffness and weakness. Osteoarthritis develops with age and normal wear and tear on the wrist but it can also develop as a result of a traumatic injury to the wrist or ligaments. The wrist is one of the first joints in the body in which arthritis naturally develops.

Rheumatoid arthritis is a systemic inflammatory disease that destroys tissues, joints and bones. Usually, rheumatoid arthritis is first detected in the smaller joints, such as the wrist and the hand.

X-rays can distinguish between various types of arthritis.

OSTEOARTHRITIS OF THE WRIST

What causes it?

- Aging
- Normal wear and tear on the wrist
- Previous injury to the forearm, wrist or ligaments

What are the symptoms?

- Pain, stiffness, swelling
- Limited motion of the wrist
- Difficulty in bending the wrist
- Diminished grip strength

What is the treatment?

- Anti-inflammatory medication
- Modify the activities that cause pain
- Immobilize the wrist with a splint for a short time to alleviate swelling and pain
- Exercise the hand to strengthen it. Consult a physician or physiotherapist to obtain the correct exercise program and technique.
- Cortisone injections
- If joint function decreases, surgery may be an option. Surgical options include removing the arthritic bone, joint fusion to make the joint solid and joint replacement.

CHAPTER 28

Shoulder Injuries

The shoulder joint is a ball and socket joint where the top of the arm bone (humerus) forms a joint with the shoulder blade (scapula). The rotator cuff is a group of four muscles and their tendons that help to control shoulder joint motion.

One muscle comes from the top of the shoulder, one from the front and two from the back. These muscles attach to the humerus by way of their tendons, which are fused together, giving them the name rotator "cuff". These muscles are used to raise the arm over the head, as well as to rotate it toward and away from the body. They help to keep the shoulder in its socket, preventing dislocation.

Above the rotator cuff is the acromion, which is a bony projection of the scapula. Between the rotator cuff tendons and the acromion is a protective fluid filled sac called the bursa. When you raise your arm, there is contact between the rotator cuff, the acromion and the bursa. A strong and healthy rotator cuff holds the humeral head down in the socket without causing upward pressure on the acromion.

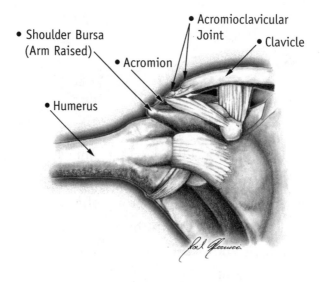

- Shoulder Bursa (Arm Raised)
- Acromioclavicular Joint
- Clavicle
- Acromion
- Humerus

ROTATOR CUFF TENDONITIS

The rotator cuff is a group of four muscles and their tendons that help to control shoulder joint motion. Rotator cuff tendonitis is an inflammation of one or more of the tendons in the shoulder. When the rotator cuff is injured, pain usually doesn't focus in one place. There will be tenderness in the shoulder area, especially if the arm is raised above shoulder level.

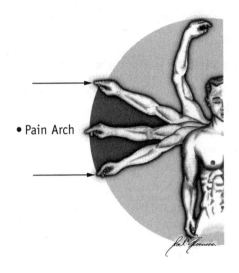

• Pain Arch

Magnetic resonance imaging (MRI) and ultrasound can be used to confirm this injury.

What Causes It?

- Repetitive overhead activities, such as tennis, basketball or baseball can injure the tendons
- A fall or accident can cause injury to the tendons
- Degeneration with aging

What Are the Symptoms?

- Dull ache in the outer arm and shoulder
- Pain at the shoulder when lifting the arm above shoulder level
- Pain may extend down to the elbow, but not beyond
- Pain is more prominent at night or when lying on the shoulder
- Cracking of the shoulder may be experienced

What is the treatment?

- Icing and resting the shoulder is important
- Stop the activity that caused the problem initially
- Anti-inflammatory drugs
- Ultrasound treatments, massage and electrical stimulation
- Most important is stretching and strengthening the rotator cuff with resistance exercise. Consult a physician or physiotherapist for the proper exercise and technique.
- If these treatments fail, cortisone injections can be made into the bursa above the tendon. No more than three injections should be given. More injections can weaken the tendon and cause it to rupture.

- For severe injuries, surgery may be required. Arthro–scopic procedures are the least invasive. A small portion of the acromiom is removed to relieve pressure on the rotator cuff.

ROTATOR CUFF TEAR

Rotator cuff tear is an injury caused by tearing one of the tendons in the rotator cuff.

Magnetic resonance imaging (MRI) and ultrasound can show if there is a tear in the tendon, or if the tendon is detached from the bone. If there is a tear in the tendon, testing can show if it is a complete tear or a partial tear.

What Causes It?

- This injury is most common in people over 40 years of age, but can occur in younger individuals after acute trauma or some repetitive sports activities. Activities that lift the arm over the head, such as in tennis, baseball, or swimming are more likely to cause this injury.
- Shoulder fracture or dislocation.

- The rotator cuff can weaken and tear in a person who has had tendonitis of the rotator cuff and did not have the injury treated.

What Are the Symptoms?

- Dull ache in the outer arm and shoulder when you lift your arm or lower it from a lifted position. You may feel pain in the front of the shoulder, radiating down the side of the arm to the elbow. At first, the pain may be noticeable after doing an over the head activity, but later it can be present at all times.
- May have stiffness and loss of motion.
- If the injury is caused by trauma, there may be an immediate acute pain, a cracking of the shoulder and a weakness in the arm.
- Wasting of muscles above the shoulder.

What is the treatment?

- Rest and ice the shoulder, and take anti-inflammatory drugs.

- Strengthening exercises and physiotherapy. Consult a physician or physiotherapist for the proper exercises and techniques. It could take many weeks or months to restore the mobility and strength of the shoulder.
- Surgical procedure may be required to suture the tear.

FROZEN SHOULDER

Frozen shoulder is a disorder that causes a thickening of the capsule of the shoulder joint. This disorder causes pain, stiffness and loss of motion of the shoulder joint. It is more common in women than in men and usually affects people in the 40 to 70 year old age group. Surgery and other medical problems such as diabetes, Parkinson's disease and cardiac disease can cause an increased risk of developing frozen shoulder.

Frozen shoulder can be confirmed using X–rays and magnetic resonance imaging (MRI).

What Causes It?

- The causes are not fully understood.

What Are the Symptoms?

- Dull aching pain, usually located over the outer shoulder and sometimes the upper arm that can last from five weeks to several months.
- Pain can ease, but stiffness and restricted motion in the shoulder remains for the next four to nine months.
- Shoulder motion slowly returns over the next six months to three years.

What Is the Treatment?

- Frozen shoulder usually gets better without intervention, but this can take up to three years.
- Anti-inflammatory medication for pain control.
- Exercise and stretching are most important to increase the motion of the joint and to minimize the loss of muscle in the affected arm. Consult a physician or physiotherapist for the proper exercises and techniques.
- A technique that I find useful is known as a "therapeutic arthrogram". This involves making an injection to the shoulder capsule of contrast material (such

as dye, air or both), followed by a small injection of cortisone. After the injection, the patient's arm is carefully manipulated to improve the range of motion.

ARTHRITIS IN ACROMIOCLAVICULAR (AC) JOINT

The AC joint is the joint in the shoulder at the point that the shoulder blade meets the collarbone. AC joint arthritis is a condition characterized by the loss of cartilage in the AC joint. As the joint wears thin, the bones begin to rub causing pain and stiffness. X-rays can be used to confirm this injury.

What Causes It?

- Aging can cause the AC joint to wear down and become inflamed. Bone spurs can form around the joint causing pressure on the muscles below.
- AC joint arthritis can appear at an earlier age in weightlifters as a result of wear and tear.
- AC joint arthritis can occur if rotator cuff problems exist.
- Previous trauma to the shoulder.

What Are the Symptoms?

- Pain and swelling with activity. Pain is usually at the top of the shoulder, but can radiate to the upper arm and the back of the shoulder.
- Reaching across the body towards the other arm can cause pain
- Sleeping on the side can cause pain
- Lifting can cause pain

What Is the Treatment?

- Rest, ice and anti–inflammatory medication.
- Cortisone injections can work to reduce swelling and pain.
- Modify activities so the condition is not aggravated. Usually, physical therapy aggravates the symptoms.
- Surgical treatment can be done with arthroscopy. A small portion of the collarbone is removed, so bones no longer rub and cause pain.

CHAPTER 29

Back Injuries

The spinal column consists of 24 bones (vertebrae), sitting one on top of each other, resting on the pelvis. At the top of the spinal column is the skull. The bones of the spine are connected to each other by discs at the front and facet joints at the back. The discs and facet joints allow the spine to bend, move and remain flexible.

The spinal cord runs through the hollow center of the spinal column. Nerve roots exit the spinal canal through small passageways between the vertebrae and the discs. Ligaments, as well as back and front body muscles, stabilize the spinal column. It is important to condition the torso muscles in order to keep the back strong and healthy.

There is a natural order in which we use our muscles when we lift, turn or move. The firing pattern is firstly, the strong gluteus muscles, then the hamstrings and finally the spinal muscles. It is important for our back health to keep these muscles firing in their natural order.

In many of the conditions that we will be discussing, the sequence has been altered, and has caused injury. Electro-myography (EMG) is a procedure that determines the order in which your muscles are firing. Once this is determined, the necessary corrections can be made by doing the proper

Examples of Disk Problems

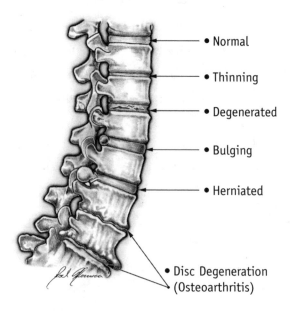

- Normal
- Thinning
- Degenerated
- Bulging
- Herniated
- Disc Degeneration (Osteoarthritis)

back strengthening exercises. The EMG scan ensures that the exercises being done are correct and effective. Each person is unique, therefore, it is necessary to be tested. Using your muscles in correct sequence keeps your back strong and healthy.

HERNIATED DISC AND BULGING DISC

A disc consists of a gel–like substance in the center (nucleus pulposus) that is surrounded by tough fibrocartilagenous fibers (annulus fibrosus). The center of the disc also contains water which helps the disc act as a shock absorber between the vertebrae.

A herniated disc occurs when there is a tear in the outer fibers, and the tear extends to the center nucleus. This tear allows the inner material to escape to the outside of the disc, and when this occurs, the nucleus material comes into contact with the spinal nerves, causing pain. A herniated disc is sometimes called a "slipped disc".

A central herniated disc is a more serious injury in which a larger amount of the nucleus material escapes from the disc putting pressure on and crushing the cauda equine nerves in the spinal cord. Depending on the size of the herniation, the nerves to both legs can be affected as well as the nerves to the bowel and bladder. This injury requires immediate attention.

In a bulging disc, the inner nucleus loses hydration which results in the disc bulging, and pressing against the nerve endings, causing pain.

Computed tomography (CT) and magnetic resonance imagery (MRI) can be used to identify if a disc has herniated and the extent of the damage.

What Causes It?

- Aging can cause the disc to dry, affecting its strength and resiliency.
- Improper lifting
- Obesity
- Smoking
- Lack of proper exercise to strengthen and protect the back
- Inadequate nutrition
- Poor posture and uncorrected spinal misalignments

What Are the Symptoms?

- Depending on where the disc has ruptured, a sudden severe pain or numbness, weakness, a tingling sensation in the arms, legs, feet, back, shoulders or neck can be experienced.

- A central herniated disc can cause loss of control of the bowel or bladder, which would require immediate medical attention.

- If the disc has herniated at the base of the spine, pain usually occurs in the lower back. Numbness may be experienced in the calf, sole of the foot, and big toe. There may be difficulty lifting the foot, walking up stairs or an inability to walk on the toes.

- A bulging disc in the lower back can cause pressure on the sciatic nerve and sharp pain will follow the nerve down the leg and into the foot. Over time, the surrounding muscles can weaken and shrink in size.

- A common cause of neck, shoulder or arm pain is a herniated cervical disc in the upper spine. Dull or sharp pain may be experienced between the shoulder blades, in the neck or radiating down the arm to the fingers. Numbness may be felt in these areas as well.

What Is the Treatment?

- Resting the back for a few days and maintaining a comfortable posture that does not cause pain, to allow the inflammation to resolve. Bed rest is not recommended as the muscles may weaken further and cause the condition to worsen.
- Exercise is vital, but must be effective and safe. It is advised to consult a physician to get the proper exercise program for your back.
- Anti-inflammatory medication.
- Epidural steroid injection with X-rays to direct the medication to the right area.
- Physical therapy using different methods, such as ultrasound, traction or electrical muscle stimulation to relax the muscles.
- Stretching or gentle massage.
- Pool therapy can ease the stress on the spinal column while still allowing muscles to be exercised.
- Surgery may be necessary, if non-invasive treatments don't help.
- Central herniated disc requires surgery to relieve pressure on the nerves.

DEGENERATIVE DISC DISEASE (DDD)

Degenerative disc disease or lumbago is the gradual degeneration of the discs between the vertebrae. Most common areas affected are the lower back and the neck areas.

Magnetic resonance imaging (MRI) can detect if the discs are degenerated.

What Causes It?

- Aging causes the cartilage to become thinner and more fragile over time. This causes the discs and facet joints in the spinal column to deteriorate. Any part of the spine can be affected. Degenerative disc disease affecting the neck area is called cervical disc disease. When the mid-back is affected, it is called thoracic disc disease, and if it affects the lower or lumbar spine, it is called lumbago.
- A twisting injury that weakens the disc, producing inflammatory proteins inside the disc.

What Are the Symptoms?

- With lumbar degenerative disc disease, pain is in the lower back and usually spreads to the buttocks and upper thighs. DDD is part of aging; by the time a person is 60 years old, disc degeneration is common. However, it is rare that lower back pain will progress and get worse. At times, the pain actually decreases and goes away. A fully degenerated disc no longer has the inflammatory proteins that cause the pain, so even though many people over 60 have degenerated discs, they don't suffer from pain.
- If the cervical disc is degenerating, dull or sharp pain can be experienced in the shoulder, upper back or neck.

What Is the Treatment?

- Anti-inflammatory medication to relieve the pain
- Oral steroids or epidurals
- Physical therapy
- Exercise, such as the hamstring stretch, low-impact aerobics and dynamic lumbar stabilizing exercises. Consult a physician or physiotherapist for exercises and proper techniques.

OSTEOARTHRITIS OF THE SPINE

Spinal arthritis is one of the most common causes of spinal pain. With this condition, the cartilage between the facet joints and the back portion of the spine begins to break down. This leads to pain and loss of flexibility.

Bone spurs can form around the facet joints and spinal vertebrae, and these spurs can press on the nerves causing pain. Bone spurs are a natural part of aging, and are not painful unless pressing against a nerve. They form as a response to joint instability and are nature's way of stabilizing the joint.

Lower back or lumbar osteoarthritis causes stiffness and pain in the lower spine. Cervical spine arthritis or neck osteoarthritis causes stiffness and pain in the upper spine, neck, shoulders, arms and head. Spinal osteoarthritis usually doesn't begin until after the age of 45, but is most common after the age of 60.

Computed tomography (CT) or magnetic resonance imaging (MRI) can confirm the diagnosis.

What Causes It?

- Trauma to the spine, such as from an accident, surgery, sports injuries or poor posture

- Long term repetitive joint use
- Aging
- Obesity, causing stress on weight bearing joints
- Genetics, having a family history of osteoarthritis and congenital defects of the joints
- The presence of other associated diseases such as rheumatoid arthritis, gout or diabetes

What Are the Symptoms?

- Back or neck pain and stiffness, especially just after waking up in the morning. The symptoms usually improve during the day and worsen again at night.
- Numbness, pain, tingling in the arms or legs and buttocks
- Weakness
- Muscle spasm
- Bowel/bladder changes

What is the treatment?

- Anti-inflammatory medication
- Low impact aerobics to control weight and to decrease stiffness

- Warm water exercises. Warm water increases circulation, eases pain and loosens stiff muscles and joints.
- Stretching exercise to build strength, flexibility and range of motion. Consult a physician or physiotherapist for the proper exercises and techniques.
- Exercise to strengthen the abdominal muscles that lend support to the spine
- Proper nutrition
- Brace or immobilize the affected area
- Avoid heavy lifting
- Physical therapy, heat, electrical stimulation to control muscle spasm and pain
- Surgery is seldom required

FACET JOINT ARTHRITIS

Facet joint arthritis is the degeneration of the cartilage that protects and cushions the facet joints. Lack of cartilage causes loss of motion, stiffness and pain. Degeneration of the facet joints can also result in the formation of synovial cysts. These are fluid–filled sacs that are benign, but can cause pain if they press against the spinal canal. X–rays can confirm the diagnosis.

What causes it?

■ Aging

What are the symptoms?

■ Low back pain, especially first thing in the morning
■ Pain when bending backwards
■ Stiffness and less flexibility in the joints

What is the treatment?

■ Stretching exercises for the hamstring muscles, hip joints and back. Consult a physician or physiotherapist for exercises and proper techniques.
■ Water therapy is a less painful exercise as the joints are unweighted in the water and do not generate as much pain
■ Anti–inflammatory medication

SPINAL STENOSIS

This is a medical condition where the spinal canal narrows and puts pressure on the spinal cord and nerves, causing pain. The spine can narrow in one or more of three areas – the space between the bones of the spine (vertebrae), the canals where nerves branch out from the spine, or the space at the center of the spine.

About 75% of the cases of spinal stenosis occur in the lower back. In most cases, the nerve that is affected is the sciatic nerve which runs along the back of the leg. This condition usually occurs in men and women over 50 years of age. Younger people can suffer from this condition if they have been born with a narrow spinal canal or if they have been injured in a car accident or sports activity.

Magnetic resonance imaging (MRI), X-rays and computed tomography (CT) can identify the problem.

What Causes It?

- Aging is the most common cause. As a person ages, joints may become larger, the tissues that support the spine can get thicker, and bone spurs (small growths) can develop on the bones and in the spinal canal.

- Arthritis can cause this condition. It wears away the cartilage that keeps the joints in place.
- A person can be born with a narrow spinal canal or with a curved spine (scoliosis).
- Injuries that dislocate the spinal canal or cause bone fragments to enter the spinal canal.
- Tumors on the spine; these abnormal growths of soft tissue can affect the spinal canal by causing inflammation or by growing into the canal.
- Fluorosis or too much fluoride in the body can lead to calcified spinal ligaments.
- Paget's disease, a chronic disorder, that results in enlarged and deformed bones.

What Are the Symptoms?

- Lower back pain that is worse when walking. Pain is lessened when bending over slightly, sometimes called the "shopping cart posture".
- Pain in the legs or arms
- Abnormal sensation in the legs, such as numbness, weakness or cramping
- Falling frequently and clumsiness

What Is the Treatment?

- Take anti-inflammatory medication to relieve swelling and pain
- Wear a brace on the lower back, especially elderly people or people with weak abdominal muscles
- Exercise, such as cycling, is recommended
- Physiotherapy. Consult with your physician or physiotherapist for the correct exercises and techniques.
- Limit activities that aggravate the pain
- If non-invasive treatments don't relieve the pain, surgery can relieve the pressure on the affected nerve.

MYOFASCIAL PAIN SYNDROME

Myofascial pain syndrome (MPS) is a chronic local or regional musculoskeletal pain disorder that can involve a muscle group or a single muscle. It is characterized by the development of myofascial trigger points that are painful when active, and refer pain to other areas of the body.

The fascia is a tough connective tissue that surrounds every muscle, bone, organ, nerve and blood vessel of the body. Therefore, a malfunction in the fascia system can cause tightening of the fascia on the muscles, nerves, organs and bones, producing intense pain.

Any active trigger point can become quiet with treatment, but can become active again with exposure to cold weather, trauma or fatigue. Also, new trigger points can arise elsewhere.

There are no laboratory tests or imaging studies that can be done to confirm the diagnosis. X-rays, computed tomography (CT) and magnetic resonance imaging (MRI) do not show the fascia.

What Causes It?

- May develop from excessive strain on a particular muscle or muscle group, ligament, tendon or bursa
- Injury to intervertebral discs
- Excessive exercise and repetitive motions can cause muscle strain
- Hormonal changes, such as menopause
- General fatigue
- Nutritional deficiencies
- Chilling of certain areas of the body, such as sitting in front of an air conditioner
- Stress or nervous tension

What Are the Symptoms?

- Local or regional pain of a stabbing, burning, aching quality
- Chronic pain
- Restricted motion of the muscle affected
- Can experience depression
- At times, can affect the nervous system, causing flushing of the skin, hypersensitivity in some areas of the skin and goose bumps
- Can experience shortness of breath

What Is the Treatment?

- Vapocoolant such as fluoromethane can be sprayed on the affected muscle and then it can be stretched slowly
- Local anesthetic can be injected into the trigger point
- Corticosteroids, saline, B12 and botulinum toxin injections can be made
- Massage therapy may help
- Acupuncture
- Exercise
- Improved nutrition
- Stress Elimination

Part V

SPIRITUALITY

CHAPTER 30

How Does Spirituality Affect Our Health?

I strongly believe that seeking, exploring, and nurturing our spirit plays a major role in our health and well-being. We cannot achieve optimal health and fitness without embracing our spirit and developing its strength and full potential. Spirituality is as vital to our health as is proper diet and exercise and should not be neglected. Nurturing our spirit contributes to our eternal well-being just as proper diet and exercise contribute to our physical well-being.

It is important to define the distinction between spirituality and religion. Since religion is man's attempt to organize a system to relate to God, it can create barriers that segregate people. Conversely, spirituality is non-confrontational and a personal experience that benefits every individual who pursues it. Spirituality cannot be defined by any religion. Cultural historian William Irwin Thompson comments that, "Religion is not identical with spirituality; rather religion is the form spirituality takes in civilization." A USA Today Gallup Poll showed that:

- About 50% considered themselves religious
- About 33% considered themselves spiritual but not religious

You can be a religious person without being spiritual. Attending a place of worship and participating in the requisite religious rites and rituals does not make you spiritual. Likewise you can be a spiritual person without being religious. Spirituality is a personal experience centered in a belief that life is more than the sensual pleasures that we experience daily in our lives. It is of no consequence if you practice one of the many religions or if you do not. You will obtain major benefits to your health by discovering, developing, nurturing and cultivating your spirit.

Nurturing your spiritual being is a continual process that requires daily exercise and maintenance, no different than exercising your muscles to maintain your physical fitness.

To ignore it for long periods of time will cause it to atrophy just as your muscles would without attention.

When you have the openness, willingness and eagerness to discover your spiritual self, then you will be amazed at how quickly the tools will be provided to you. An ancient Taoist saying states, "When you are ready to learn, the teacher will appear." You will see the teacher and the lesson only when you are truly eager and ready to learn it, otherwise you will continue on your current path. Without action our faith will become forgotten and fade away. You must study and remain interested and inquisitive and continue to persevere to find the path that is right for you. When you embark on this exploration, then your soul will come alive and you will find a calmness that you have never experienced before.

For me, spirituality is that divine gift which connects me to God. While many religions believe in a deity that dwells within every person, I reiterate that you don't have to be religious to be spiritual.

I grew up as a Christian in a Catholic family and even though I would attend church regularly, my thoughts while at church were not always on God. In my teens I decided on a career in medicine and soon my technical learning overpowered my faith. With my scientific mind I explained away spirituality as something that did not exist. I could not prove it existed, so it didn't. I had drifted completely away from religion and God and focused only on establishing my career in medicine.

I believe my spiritual awakening began in May 2001. I had endured three sleepless nights with only one thought on my mind, and that was Jerusalem and a strong desire to visit that city. I had no explanation for this sudden powerful and overwhelming desire to go there, but the urge was so strong that a week later I was on a plane headed for Jerusalem. On my arrival, I visited the Church of the Nativity. I spent several hours there on my own. I thought of nothing in particular but for the first time in years I felt very much at peace and enjoyed the feeling.

I wandered about the Old City of Jerusalem for several days before finding a small chapel, Dominus Flevit, on The Mount of Olives. For the next week, I felt a need to spend several hours a day there. I enjoyed the peace I felt and was content spending time on my own. One day, my thoughts turned to imagining how incredible it would be to attend a mass in this chapel. I thought how much more meaningful it would be for me now, unlike the many times I attended mass as a youngster when I was feeling no connection to God. At this moment, after days of not seeing a soul in this chapel, a group from Italy walked in, saw me sitting on my own and asked me if I would like to participate in mass.

This mass was extremely meaningful to me and I attained a level of peace and contentment that I had never before experienced. My passion to find out more about God was ignited. I could only describe what I felt as experiencing an intravenous injection of a combination of love and fire coursing through me, giving me a strong desire to understand and investigate this joyful occurrence.

I know now that this was the time of my spiritual awakening. Jerusalem has been considered the Holy City by Jews, Christians and Muslims for centuries, so it did not surprise me that I was called to this place to begin my spiritual journey. While others have pursued various different pathways in their spiritual quest, my own journey took me back to my Christian roots, and I found my connection with God through a renewal of my faith, not through conforming to religious requirements.

When I returned home, I relentlessly searched for everything I could find out about God, the history, the purpose, my quest giving birth to more questions than answers. I continued to find my medical practice stimulating, but I also passionately wanted to explore my renewed spirituality. I have been back to Jerusalem many times since that first visit and my desire to nurture my spirit has become ever more compelling. I know now that this is an essential part of my well-being.

I realized that I had been concentrating on healing the physical side of my patients, but now I believe this is not enough. My own experience proved this to me. I had felt the change. The physical side, the part we can see and measure, is but a small portion of our overall well-being. To obtain complete health, we have to address our spiritual being, the part we can't see or measure but that actually represents the major part of our wellness. While the body is only temporary, the spirit is eternal.

I believe that every person possesses a divinely created spirit with the innate capacity and capability of connecting with the divine. However, many are unaware of this or refuse to acknowledge its existence. Our spirit is a gift that we have received from our Creator. It is our divine link to God. It's a way of making a connection to and developing a relationship with God. We must strive to nurture this component as it is an essential part of our being. Furthermore, we cannot consider ourselves totally healthy without it.

A significant amount of research has been done on near death experiences. A typical experience almost always mentions pleasant feelings of calmness and peace, a sensation of moving upwards through a tunnel and encountering a Being of Light. Most people are reluctant to return to the here and now preferring to stay and enjoy this state of peace and calmness. Whenever God, saints and spiritual beings are pictured, they are bathed in an aura of intense light.

We are all given this divine precious light, a divinely created spirit with the capacity to connect with God, but initially it is but a tiny flicker within us. We must seek it and nourish it, and work on it to help it develop so it can shine with intensity. Many of us push it to the recesses of our being where we are no longer aware of its existence and some totally reject it. We must bring it to the forefront. We should let our light shine so that others may see this light being reflected through our lives. Our spirit connects us with the divine and separates us from the material world and it is only after we strengthen this bond that we can attain peace and contentment.

Many times we ignore our spirit until our life is in crisis, such as when we are confronted with illness or death. It is important for us not to wait for a critical time in our lives to find God. We must learn to seek spirituality at the time that we are not in crisis and this will help to promote wellness.

We have many distractions in our busy lives. We plod along in a certain direction, distracted by promises and temptations, engrossed in everyday struggles. Sometimes, we become guided by greed and obsessed with accumulating possessions and material gains. Negative thoughts and feelings take over and we lose the contentment and joy of living because of the many pressures. At times, we attain our wanted achievements and still we feel like something is missing. We are not at peace.

Spirituality is an important part of a person's health and well-being. Our physical health cannot reach its full potential without having our spiritual health in place. We need to investigate, understand and feed our spirit. As we pursue this process, our overall health will improve.

All who believe tend to fare better in every aspect of their life, be it health, emotional well-being, or worldly success. If our spirit is neglected, every area of our lives will be adversely affected.

How does spirituality result in health benefits? When the body is relaxed, the breathing rate, blood pressure and heart rate go down thus decreasing stress. When the nervous system is not under stress, the immune system functions better. Studies indicate that spiritual people heal faster, have less illness, feel less pain, have lower cortisol levels and live longer. Research also shows that comfort and strength is gained from spirituality which contributes to healing and the sense of well-being.

The closer you draw to spirituality, the closer you are to reaching optimal health. You will be at total peace with yourself and anxiety will not exist. As our spirituality grows, we will find that reality changes for the better.

Spirituality is a powerful entity that goes far beyond proper nutrition and exercise. Exercising the spirit requires as much work, if not more work, than exercising the body. We cannot achieve perfect health without attending to our spirit.

Often we will buy a book on exercise with great intentions to work on getting our body into shape, but we lose interest and never do the exercises. We cannot achieve physical fitness without doing any of the exercises. Just reading the book is not enough. We must practice the behavior and actually feel it before we receive the benefits.

When trying to improve our fitness level, we often are sidetracked by new and improved exercise plans and new ways of losing weight that are easier and faster. We might find it difficult to stay motivated and on course as we are bombarded by these temptations. Similarly, we will have distractions and temptations on our way to achieving spiritual health. We must work at it and stay motivated to improve and enjoy the plentiful benefits.

Spiritual growth helps us connect with God through meditation and prayer, and God communicates with us through our feelings and intuition. When we develop openness to spiritual growth, we find coincidences and synchronicity all around us. We ask and then we listen. Our answers come to us in the form of human connection, books, a conversation or even a song. As you strengthen your relationship with God, you are rewarded with increased awareness, deeper insights and stronger faith and hope in your life. Your life becomes worry-free and your stress level drops. Spiritual growth provides the tools to help your life flow more harmoniously. You become more attuned to your greater purpose.

Many teaching tools are available. Prayer and meditation are exercises of the spirit and are ways of developing our spiritual health. There are many works of literature that are helpful. When you are ready and eager to learn, ask God for guidance and then the resources needed will begin to present themselves.

We need to continually practise and exercise the lessons that we learn. We must continue to work on the reconciliation of our spirit with God. Everyone needs to be reconnected and reconciled with God to find peace and joy. Knowing the theory is not enough. It must be put to use and practiced so that it becomes second nature.

To achieve happiness we must achieve a balance in our lives. We get distracted as to what is important, the innocence, excitement, passion, purity, love and righteousness. God works from the inside out. Spirituality is man's ability to connect with God and to be indwelt by God, and then to reflect a divine nature of God through the renewed human spirit. When we look at a spiritual person we see

God's divine light being reflected in this person. It is this light that connects us to each other, to the universe and to God. Our health as individuals and the health of all nations depends on it.

The spirit is the non-physical part of every human being that never ages. If we fill our thoughts with faith and getting to a place where we are incapable of envy, jealousy, vengeance and hate, we will reach a more relaxed and satisfied state.

By striving to feed our spiritual self, we have a deeper appreciation for life and all that it has to offer. Our spirituality will flow to those around us, and guide them and us towards peace, contentment, joyfulness and optimal health.

Afterword

I hope you have enjoyed reading *Dr. Galea's Secrets to Optimal Health – Body and Spirit*. In the first 29 chapters of my book, I have given you pertinent information that you need to improve your physical and mental health. While this is important – to concentrate on, and obsess over, our physical and mental wellness, will not bring us optimal health. I believe the most dramatic and life-changing secret to optimal health is found in Chapter 30. We must put our main focus on discovering and healing our spiritual self.

Index